Missing Factor
A Personal Experience of Haemophilia

By Marie Berger

Missing Factor
A Personal Experience of Haemophilia

By Marie Berger

Published by
Chipmunkapublishing
PO Box 6872
Brentwood
Essex CM13 1ZT
United Kingdom

First published 2005

A record of this book is in the British Library.

Printing sponsored by RPM Print & Design,
www.rpm-repro.co.uk

ISBN 1-904697-74-7

http://www.chipmunkapublishing.com

To my children

Simon, Rachel, Nathan, Benjamin and Joel

Acknowledgements

Thanks are due to staff at the Haemophilia Society (UK), in particular Anna Hinchliffe-Wood, Ruth Taylor and John Morris, for their enormous help and encouragement. I am grateful also, to the following for giving generously of their time and providing me with a wealth of information:- Doctor Mark Adelman, consultant haematologist at Lincoln County Hospital Haemophilia Centre; Kate Khair, nurse consultant at Great Ormond Street Paediatric Haemophilia Centre; Carol Martin, clinical nurse specialist at Leicester Comprehensive Care Centre; Lorraine Birtwistle, haemophilia nurse specialist at Manchester Comprehensive Care Centre. Finally, but no less importantly, my thanks to Les, my husband, for his invaluable computer skills, his many helpful suggestions and his patience throughout the writing of this book.

Contents

Foreword

Being told that your child has a chronic inherited condition is possibly one of the worst things a new parent can hear. Haemophilia causes internal bleeding, particularly into joints and in cases of severe haemophilia this bleeding can occur spontaneously for no obvious reason. A diagnosis may mean regular infusions of factor VIII or IX, trips to the hospital and that some activities, particularly high impact sports such as rugby and karate, should be avoided. Having a child diagnosed with haemophilia will undoubtedly have a huge effect on your life. However, the reality is that modern medicine means that most young people with haemophilia can lead a relatively 'normal' life. The Haemophilia Society hears from many young adults with bleeding disorders that have gone on to travel the world or been to university and lead fulfilled lives. This is not to say that they have not encountered difficulties on the way, which is why this book is so important.

This book is written by the mother of a now grown-up boy with haemophilia and is a follow up to her first book 'Understanding Haemophilia' published in 1989. It deals with all the challenges and successes a parent of a child with haemophilia can expect to encounter, Marie's practical insights will serve as a resource for parents in dealing with haemophilia in the family setting and also within the medical profession.

In this book Marie details her experiences of haemophilia from the time of diagnosis all the way into adulthood. Reading about Marie's encounters may provide you with answers to the many questions you will undoubtedly have. By sharing in someone else's experiences you should also be reassured that you are not as isolated as you may feel and that others have felt the way that you do now.

This book will also guide you through the additional milestones of a child with haemophilia such as the first bleed, starting home treatment and beginning school.

Marie's book shows that having a child with haemophilia need not destroy your life and the dreams you have for your family. This is a positive book, which charts the course of a child growing up into adolescence and adulthood; how to cope when they want to do sports or activities that keep you awake at night worrying, letting go and allowing them to grow up and take responsibility for their haemophilia.

This is a book that you will no doubt return to over the years whenever haemophilia causes concern or questions. It should provide you with answers and a starting place for resolving any problems you encounter.

Anna Hinchliffe-Wood
Children & youth worker
The Haemophilia Society

Preface

When I was pregnant for the first time, I was terrified at the thought of having anything wrong with my baby. 'I'd have to leave it in the hospital,' I said. 'There's no way I could cope...'

*   *   *

When haemophilia is first diagnosed, the relatives of a sufferer are often too shocked to ask many questions. And when they told me that my son Nathan had haemophilia I just stood there, unable to take it in. Fear and shock block the channels of receptiveness at that stage . . . we may ask a lot of questions, but we do not hear the answers.

I know how frightening haemophilia can be at first and how that fear can be made worse by sensational remarks in the media, like: 'Haemophiliacs can bleed to death after a small cut'. This simply isn't true, yet because it's in the papers or on the television, people believe it. The obvious person to consult about this medical condition should be your doctor. However, most GPs are never presented with a case of haemophilia for diagnosis. Their knowledge of it is largely limited to a few lectures on the subject at medical school and any cases they saw as junior hospital doctors.

This book is an attempt to give the sort of information that I should have liked at my finger-tips when Nathan was first diagnosed . . . the shared experience of the trauma of diagnosis . . . clear, straightforward answers to the sort of questions that any parent might ask on discovering that their child has haemophilia. First and foremost, it is intended to inform and reassure parents of a child with a bleeding disorder, some of whom may still be trying to deal with the emotional aftermath of diagnosis. I hope it will also interest those who enjoy the insight and understanding to be gained from a personal experience story.

For the sake of convenience, the word 'he' is generally used in the book when referring to a person with haemophilia. This in no way intended to be sexist. It is just that the English language is limited in this respect! Having brought up five children, including a son with severe haemophilia and a daughter who carries the gene, I am familiar with the ups and downs of living with this condition. But I know too that it is perfectly possible not just to cope with a blood disorder but to have a normal, happy family life where haemophilia has ceased to be a dominating factor.

CHAPTER ONE

Hidden Handicap

Birth

'You've got a little boy!' I sank back onto the bed, utterly drained, but relieved that the long labour was finally over. Les, my husband, put his arm round me. 'Well done, love,' he whispered. From the tightly wrapped bundle that the midwife placed beside me peered two small dark eyes in a red, wrinkled face, much of it covered by a fine, black down. I kissed the tiny snub nose. Nathan was beautiful. Nervously I loosened the blanket, checked limbs, fingers, toes ... he was perfect. I put him to my breast and he began sucking straight away, creating an immediate closeness between us.

Weighing eight pounds and twelve ounces, Nathan passed every medical check for new-borns before he left hospital and our other children, six-year-old Simon and three-year-old Rachel, were delighted with their baby brother.

On the move

We all enjoyed the milestones of early babyhood - Nathan's first gummy smile, his responsive gurgling noises, the day he rolled over, the first time he sat up unaided, his first tooth. Then, at eight months, he began to crawl. One evening, undressing him at bath time, I noticed several nasty-looking bruises on both his knees. Deep purple, raised in the centre, they stretched the skin until it was shiny. We were puzzled, unable to connect them with any incident.

The more active Nathan became, the more bruises we counted - on knees, elbows and forehead.' Some children do bruise easily,' our doctor reassured us. But, a few days later, when a discoloured lump appeared on Nathan's chest I rang the surgery again. 'Don't worry,' said the doctor, 'There's not a lot of flesh there, so it looks much worse.' Fearing I might be branded an over-anxious mother, I did nothing about the bruise, like black, spreading paint, on Nathan's bottom and tried to ignore the semi-permanent bump on his forehead – a result of tumbles as he toddled about. Mustn't fuss. The doctor would know if something was wrong.

But the suspicious glances whenever I took Nathan out made me feel uncomfortable, almost guilty. 'Looks as though I've been battering him, doesn't it?' I remarked lightly in response to one particularly accusing stare when I was waiting outside the school gates to collect Simon and Rachel. As I ruffled Nathan's curly hair, he smiled up at me. It hurt me to see those bruises on his cheek and forehead, to accept that he really did look like a battered child. When he was eighteen months old Nathan fell, cutting his fraenum - the piece of skin inside the mouth that joins the lip to the gum. It never seemed to stop bleeding, starting again whenever Nathan sucked his thumb. Several Dracula-like grins from Nathan convinced us that he needed medical help. In Casualty, the doctor put in a stitch to solve the problem. 'It often bleeds a lot there,' he said.

Crisis point

At twenty-one months Nathan was a happy lively toddler with a friendly nature and an irrepressible sense of fun. I was six months pregnant, feeling healthy and contented. One Sunday morning he cried when he bumped his leg on the small table that he had converted into a pretend car. A kiss and cuddle seemed to make it better, but a few hours later Nathan limped to me in obvious distress. The calf muscle of his left leg was swollen, rock hard and painful to the touch.

We rang our G.P. for an urgent appointment, convinced that he would know what was causing the swelling. I felt the first stirrings of panic when he frowned, sighed and then suggested we take Nathan to hospital. 'What's the matter? Is he going to be all right?' My voice shook. Being pregnant, I was more vulnerable than usual to any crisis.

The doctor shook his head. 'He's possibly got a blood infection ... I just don't know what's wrong.'

Trying to determine the cause

That Sunday evening in our local hospital they took X-rays. Nothing was broken. A doctor examined Nathan from head to toe. 'Is there any history of blood disorders?' Les and I knew of none. With Nathan in pain and unable to walk it was difficult to remain calm. We kept hearing scraps of conversation about him outside our cubicle.

'Leukaemia. . . Christmas disease . . .'We grew more and more anxious. 'We don't know what's wrong with Nathan,' said the paediatrician. 'We'd like to admit him for tests. You can stay with him,' he added kindly. In the children's ward Nathan cried bitterly as the doctor took a blood sample.

Afterwards, when drugs lessened the pain in his leg, he fell asleep. I was so relieved when, later, a doctor told me that blood tests had eliminated some serious problems like leukaemia. He said it was likely that Nathan had a mild clotting deficiency which, it was hoped, would clear up on its own, without treatment. And I was able to sleep.

However, the following morning there was something terribly wrong – the swelling had spread downwards to Nathan's ankle and foot. That Monday afternoon we were taken to Addenbrookes, in Cambridge, a large teaching hospital with highly sophisticated blood-testing equipment.

Treating the symptoms

The more formal atmosphere of Addenbrookes, with its interminable maze of corridors, seemed forbidding after our friendly local hospital. Nathan was whisked away from me into a curtained room. His persistent screams of 'Mummy!' cut through me as I waited impatiently outside. When I was finally allowed in the doctor explained that they needed a lot of blood and it had been a slow process gathering it drip by drip from Nathan's unaffected foot. Seeing the little tear-stained face, I was unable to hold back my emotions and I cried, holding him close.

Nathan was admitted later that day. I was grateful for the many kindnesses shown me by other mothers whose own children were seriously ill. They made me cups of tea, listened sympathetically to my concerns about Nathan and offered to play with him while I snatched some much-needed rest.

Just before midnight a doctor informed me that the first tests showed some deficiency in Nathan's blood-clotting mechanism, but they had not yet managed to isolate the problem. To prevent further bleeding they would have to set up a plasma drip that would supply everything needed to clot Nathan's blood. I was welcomed into the treatment room by a doctor who believed that babies are happier with mum around. Nathan whimpered, but this time he did not scream; I was able to comfort him ... it was considerably less traumatic than the earlier experience.

The bombshell

Tuesday morning: Nathan played happily in his cot. Although still unable to stand, he was free of pain and, since the swelling had lessened slightly, I was optimistic that he would make a complete recovery. It was mid-morning when the consultant paediatrician appeared, surrounded by junior doctors, nurses and students.

He came straight to the point. 'We've now got the full results of yesterday's blood tests. I'm sorry to tell you, but your son has severe haemophilia.' He sounded so matter-of-fact, so casual. For him, the diagnosis was part of a day's work. For me, it felt like a death sentence . . . haemophilia - didn't that mean you could bleed to death from the slightest cut? For a moment, it was as if everything froze: white coated figures, their backs to the window, watching me. I was stunned . . .

speechless . . . Suddenly, so many questions. 'What about my unborn baby? Will it be affected?'

I spread one hand protectively over my stomach. The consultant laughed. 'We'd have to do a Caesarean Section on you to find out at this stage.' 'I just want to know the genetic implications,' I said tersely. He looked uneasy. 'You'd have to consult a genetic counsellor about that,' he said, already moving towards the door.

I phoned Les. 'Nathan's got haemophilia,' I managed to say between sobs. Silence. 'Are they sure?' There was a painful lump in my throat: 'Yes.' A few minutes later, he rang me back. 'Dad said that when he took lots of aspirin he had some dreadful nose bleeds,' he said reassuringly.

That was it! We had been dosing Nathan with Disprin for a heavy cold. I approached the ward sister, convinced that this vital piece of information would change the diagnosis. 'Wouldn't make a great deal of difference,' she said.

The aftermath

Dazed, I wandered back to Nathan's cot and stared out of the window . . . people driving in or out of the car park, people walking, smiling, chatting and behaving normally. Why hadn't their world stopped when mine did? I was numbed, incapable of coherent thought and could only nod in response to kind words and endless cups of tea. A young woman doctor sat down beside me.

'What about the Disprin?' I tried weakly. 'It might have worsened the situation,' she said gently, 'but it wouldn't have caused it. Your son has always had haemophilia. I'll try to answer all your questions, but you probably won't remember many of the answers,' she added kindly.

She was right. When there were no more questions I knew only that my Nathan had a serious life-long condition for which there was no known cure. 'It's like losing a loved one,' she said. 'You need to grieve.' I picked up Nathan, his face framed by a mass of curly, black hair. Cuddling him, I released some of the terrible pain. He fingered my tears, looking up at me, his deep brown eyes puzzled. 'Mummy cry,' he said.

Floundering for a way to cope

Going home was traumatic. In hospital Nathan had seemed safe while he played on my lap or slept in his cot. How could I possibly hope to protect him from the many hazards of an active toddler's day? Yet I was determined to try. Had he been made of priceless bone china, he could not have been more cosseted. To avoid the vice-like tightening in my head whenever Nathan fell as he played with the other children, I devised numerous sitting down games for him. I carried him with me when I did the housework and put him to bed extra early each evening. I reassured myself that while he was asleep he couldn't come to any harm.

'You'll have to stop this,' said Les. 'You're getting neurotic. He'll be more at risk if you never let him do anything.' And Les coped far better. He took Nathan out for walks to escape my stifling over-protectiveness, strengthened his muscles by the exercise and laid the foundation of their relationship. To take me away from my son during the day I accepted an offer of supply teaching. I had begun to fear my own child - he personified this awful thing that had invaded our lives. Nathan and haemophilia were synonymous.

Then some of my anger emerged with the tears. Why him? Why us? I raged. We'd done nothing to deserve this. Rage followed by guilt. Perhaps Nathan's haemophilia resulted from something I had done in pregnancy. Was it some sort of divine retribution for past wrong doings? The future loomed dismally for all of us. Maybe Nathan would not outlive his childhood. Or, if he did, this cruel blood disorder might cripple him.

My fears were intensified by well-meant phone calls. Other parents of haemophilic children, who had been put in touch with me by the hospital, told me their own frightening experiences, stories of horrific disasters. 'I'm so sorry,' said the voice on the other end of the line. 'We've been through hell on earth with Christopher.' 'But Nathan was almost two before we found out.' I said, 'so perhaps it will be different.'

'You've got to face up to reality,' I was told. It seemed that their children had also known occasional problems at this stage. But, with time, the number of 'bleeds' increased dramatically. 'Bleeds' is one of the new words I had to learn to live with. On the premise that knowing your enemy is half the battle, I started to find out all I could about haemophilia. I read every book I could find, talked to doctors and joined the London-based Haemophilia Society. The future now seemed slightly less bleak.

CHAPTER TWO

About Haemophilia

What is it?

Haemophilia is a defect of the blood that inhibits normal clotting. The word derives from the Greek: haima, blood and philia, loving or fond - meaning that the person affected by it appears to love blood, which is ironic, because fear is the usual reaction to loss of blood. This blood-clotting disorder is congenital, lifelong and at present there is no cure. There are three main hereditary bleeding disorders: haemophilia A; haemophilia B (or Christmas disease, named after the first patient in whom it was discovered); and Von Willebrand's Disease, named after the Swedish doctor who discovered it; other varieties are extremely rare. The most common type, haemophilia A, is also known as classical haemophilia. Some people refer to haemophilia as a disease. However, disease is usually associated with ideas of 'illness' or 'contagion', neither of which applies. So I prefer the words: condition, disability, or blood disorder.

How do you get it?

Haemophilia is the result of an abnormal gene. In thirty percent of cases there is no known family history. And an extremely unusual condition known as 'acquired haemophilia' may occur apparently spontaneously, mainly in the middle-aged and elderly. It happens when the patient's own immune system has developed antibodies that attack the body's supply of Factor VIII, a vital blood-clotting protein.

With a known family history the transmission of haemophilia may be anticipated. But in some cases, such as where a parent was adopted as a child, the link might not be known. At conception each of us has between fifty thousand and one hundred thousand genes, half from the mother and half from the father.

Genes are minute threads of material that are attached to chromosomes in every cell of the body and they come in pairs. They tell our bodies precisely how to function and determine exactly what we look like. For example: blue or brown eyes, big or little nose, dark or fair hair. Chromosomes are the bundles of matter that carry these genes. Females have two X-chromosomes, so called because under microscopes they look that shape. Males, on the other hand, have an X and a Y chromosome.

It is the male who determines the sex of any children: if the X-chromosome in the female egg joins up with a Y chromosome in the male sperm, the result will be a boy; if the male passes on an X chromosome, the resulting two Xs will make a girl. Sometimes genes mutate. These changes are then passed on from one generation to another. In other words, they are inherited. Seven out of ten people with haemophilia have a family history of the disorder; new genetic changes account for the remainder.

Because haemophilia is only carried on the X-chromosome, none of the sons of a man with haemophilia will be affected by the disability, since they have all inherited a Y-chromosome from him. But all his daughters will be carriers because they carry his X-chromosome.

As the severity of the condition usually passes on unaltered, a person with severe haemophilia will transmit severe haemophilia, a moderately affected sufferer moderate haemophilia, a mildly affected person a mild form. Daughters of men with haemophilia usually do not themselves suffer from the condition – if they do, it will be a mild form. The normal X gene on the chromosome from their mother usually protects them by making enough of the missing clotting factor. They do, however, have a fifty-fifty chance of giving birth to haemophilic sons and the same probability of their own daughters being carriers.

In the unusual event of a haemophilic male marrying a carrier there is a fifty-fifty chance of any daughters or sons having haemophilia. If their haemophilic daughter in her turn has children, all her sons will have haemophilia and all daughters will be carriers. There are three types of carrier: the daughter of a man with haemophilia; the sister of a boy with the condition; and the mother of a newly-diagnosed son where there is no known history. Queen Victoria was a carrier of haemophilia; and her two daughters were carriers. Through a daughter and grandchild the gene for haemophilia spread to the Russian and Spanish Royal families. However, as her son King Edward VII had not inherited the faulty gene his descendants were unaffected. To sum up: All the daughters of a person with haemophilia will be carriers but none of his sons will be carriers or have haemophilia; a carrier daughter has a fifty-fifty chance of having haemophilic sons and carrier daughters. And sometimes it can occur in a previously unaffected family.

Clotting

In haemophilia there is no normal blood-clotting. The clotting process is complex. Whenever we cut or bruise ourselves, an intricate process begins, which results in a clot forming at the site of injury. Blood flows from a damaged blood vessel and triggers off a chain reaction between different elements in the blood, which all play an important part in the clotting process. How many of these elements are involved to stop bleeding depends on the severity of the injury.

When a small blood vessel is injured, as in a pinprick, the walls of that vessel contract; this temporarily stops the bleeding. This first aid is then continued by the platelets, tiny pieces in the blood that are able to stick together and form a plug. This gives time for the clotting factors to work together to solidify blood into a clot, which seals the wound properly. There are twelve known clotting factors, which are numbered in the Roman way.

People with haemophilia A have a lack of Factor VIII in their blood, whereas those suffering from Christmas disease, haemophilia B, are deficient in factor IX. Haemophilias A and

B manifest themselves in much the same way, but Von Willebrand's Disease creates a variety of different problems since there is a deficiency of a plasma factor which impairs platelet function as well as in most cases a lack of Factor VIII.

Most of the clotting factors are proteins, nutritional substances in the body, many of which are made in the liver. Although Factor VIII is produced in the liver, it is also made in other places such as the spleen, kidneys and blood vessel walls. Each of the twelve clotting factors must act on cue for the effective production of a clot. But why not simply one factor to make a clot? Because if, in seconds, a massive amount of one factor stopped blood flow, it could drastically interfere with the functions of vital parts of the body like heart, lungs and brain. Clotting occurs after a controlled, steady process which has inbuilt fail-safe mechanisms.

This process is activated when a blood vessel is injured. The blood leaking out into surrounding tissues produces emergency signals in turn for each factor in the bloodstream. The first to act is Factor III, which, by mixing in with the blood flow, then stirs factor VII into action. Next are Factors XII and XI, which are triggered off by collagen - a substance in the lining of the blood vessel. Factor IX is now stimulated into action followed by Factor VIII and so on until Factor I completes the process of clotting.

Fortunately each factor is equipped with what has been described as a 'safety cap', which can only be removed, by another factor or chemical. It cannot merely drop off and release the factor accidentally. The normal time from wounding to coagulation is four to eight minutes. In the person with haemophilia this time is prolonged owing to insufficient Factor VIII or IX.

The activity level of Factors VIII and IX can be measured from a sample of blood in the laboratory. The normal range is wide. During pregnancy, or after injury, the body produces more of a clotting factor to cope with the unusual situation.

When the crisis is over, the level slowly decreases again. The body then has to start making more.

There is a twelve-hour half-life for Factor VIII; this means that a reading of its maximum activity in the blood will drop to a half twelve hours later, twelve hours further on will show a level of a quarter...People with mild haemophilia have between six per cent and twenty-five per cent of Factor VIII activity in their blood. Moderately affected sufferers have from one to five per cent, while those with severe haemophilia have below one per cent. They cannot make more than this. There may however be a marked discrepancy between clinical severity and the experience of haemophilic bleeds.

Bleeds

When referring to a 'bleed' we are using the literal meaning of the word - leaking blood. However, since most haemophilic problems arise in joints and muscles, much of the bleeding takes place internally beneath the skin, remaining unseen. If anyone injures a blood vessel some blood loss occurs before clotting. In a person with haemophilia blood flows no faster than normal, but lack of Factor VIII means that it may continue leaking without treatment. Haemophilic bleeding normally first occurs some time after an affected baby begins to walk, when falls and bumps are more likely.

An early sign of haemophilia is the frequent appearance of nasty-looking bruises, raised in the centre. With this sort of bruise bleeding, although continuing beyond the normal time, will finally stop when the pressure of blood from the injury equalises the pressure from surrounding body tissues. However, it is important to obtain medical advice – no sign of possible haemophilia should ever be ignored. Scratches and small cuts are rarely problematic; since minute blood vessels, capillaries, shut down to stop bleeding. They may, however, ooze longer than normal, but gentle, firm pressure on the wound will stop the bleeding. There are two important bonuses: you feel that you have some element of control and your child is confident that you are able to deal calmly with the situation.

Types of Bleeds

An important aspect of haemophilic bleeds is the need for early treatment: to stop the bleeding, to prevent severe pain and avoid the permanent damage that can result if bleeds are left untreated. Most bleeds are internal - into joints and muscles. Since these parts take the strain of many of our movements this is hardly surprising. When bleeds into one particular joint become habitual, it is termed a "target joint" and arthritis can develop.

In time, your child will be able to recognize when a bleed has started long before there is any visible sign. 'What it's like, Mummy,' Nathan told me, 'is a sort of pins and needles feeling.' The build up is gradual, so it was often a couple of hours before he complained of pain in an affected joint or muscle. 'It's a sort of sharp stabbing pain.'

When haemophilia was first diagnosed in Nathan, I worried: 'Will there be internal bleeds which perhaps I won't know about...?' 'What about bleeding into the skull with possible brain damage...?' 'Will my child end up crippled...?'

Then I learned that a person with haemophilia is no more likely to bleed into the brain than anyone else; after serious injury to the head anybody can bleed internally.

Someone who has haemophilia bleeds no faster than anyone else so provided treatment is sought promptly there is no more likelihood of permanent damage. Vomiting blood sounds frightening. But it often means simply that some blood from the back of the nose has been swallowed, irritating the stomach and causing the vomiting. Blood from the stomach might also be excreted from the bowel, turning faeces black. However, oral iron treatment can also colour the faeces.

Blood in urine generally indicates injury or inflammation, usually due to infection of the kidney, bladder, or urethra. Certain foods and medication can also colour urine red - beetroot, for example. It only takes a little blood to redden urine ... it invariably looks worse than it actually is. Whilst any internal bleeding of this sort requires medical advice and perhaps treatment, it is rarely serious.

Bleeding from deep cuts can be temporarily stemmed with pressure until treatment is available. Nose bleeds, which can happen to anyone, although alarming to look at as there seems to be a lot of blood, often stop with the standard first aid treatment of pinching the nose below the bridge. As with any child, frequent nose bleeds need a visit to the doctor. Apparently spontaneous bleeds in people with severe haemophilia are probably triggered by some injury too trivial to be noticed.

Unpredictability

You might expect someone with the lowest level of Factor VIII in their blood to always have a greater number of bleeds than a person with moderate or mild haemophilia. But this condition defies logic. One of the few predictable features of haemophilia is its unpredictability! There is no clear idea how often an affected child will require injections of the missing clotting factor. Nathan's can be several days, weeks or even months apart. As a young child he sometimes needed an injection after a bleed into his ankle during a play session in the garden, when similar activity a week earlier caused no problem.

It is obvious that overprotection is useless, since, whatever precautions we take; a bleed cannot always be prevented. There are people with haemophilia who have a tendency to seasonal bleeds, perhaps enjoying a bleed-free summer before coping with them in the autumn. There is, as yet, no widely-accepted explanation why this should be. Perhaps there is a connection between haemophilic bleeds and state of mind: in the summer your child might be more relaxed, happier, playing outdoors, going on holiday. Also, all-important exercise for strengthening joints and muscles is easier in the warmer weather.

To sum up: Haemophilia affects each child differently; a child may or may not have a recognisable pattern of bleeds; or again, a particular pattern might suddenly change. If other parents give frightening accounts of what happened to their child. . .

'When my Tommy was three, he fell head over heels down the stairs, gashed his head open, screamed and screamed and had to be rushed to hospital...'

. . . just remind yourself that your child might not have those problems.

CHAPTER THREE

Myths and Realities

Fear

Franklin D. Roosevelt said: 'The only thing we have to fear is fear itself.' Fear is rooted in the unknown. Mistakes and misconceptions can worry us. From listening to and believing them we can easily fall into a descending spiral of fear, depression and inability to cope.

There are myths about haemophilia such as:

'If your child cuts himself, he'll bleed to death.'
'Your child will grow out of it.'
'Anyone who has haemophilia will gush like a fountain if they cut themselves...'

But we can familiarise ourselves with the truth about this condition. Then we can correct or turn a deaf ear to these untruths.

'Pools of blood'

This life force arouses strong primeval emotion . . . we respond with fear, fascination, awe and respect to this richly-coloured liquid that constantly feeds every cell in the body. Belief in its beneficial effects dates back to ancient times - Egyptians bathed in it and Romans drank it in the hope that, by so doing, they could absorb the health-giving, rejuvenating properties they were sure it contained. To them blood was like ocean tides ebbing and flowing throughout the body, carrying with it the basic characteristics of personality.

The idea persisted until the beginning of the seventeenth century, when William Harvey discovered that the heart pumped blood continuously around the body. Practically all other knowledge about the blood remained unknown until the twentieth century. Although blood transfusions to save lives are now routine, the fears surrounding its flow out of the body still affect us -there are those who still believe that some of its owner's personality goes with it, that its loss might never be replaced.

There are some who fear to give or receive blood. Some people even faint at the sight of blood. Given the mysticism attached to blood, it is not surprising that legends have sprung up about blood-clotting problems. Yet the components of haemophilic blood, with the exception of one tiny, missing protein, are the same as everyone else's - red cells, white cells, platelets and plasma. Blood will flow from a cut in the person with haemophilia at the normal rate, no more, no less. When firm pressure is applied to the wound, bleeding will stop long enough for medical help to be obtained. So this type of drama is extremely unlikely.

'Bleeding to death from a tiny cut without medical intervention'

Bleeding from tiny cuts, as I have previously explained, usually presents no problem whatsoever - apart from the nuisance value involved in extended oozing time. But it is understandable that, without knowledge of the true nature of haemophilia, people might think that life presents constant dangers for a person with the condition . . . one scratch, with no immediate medical help, resulting in probable death. Indeed, this was my belief at the time of Nathan's diagnosis. 'What if he gets a bad cut?' I used to say to Les. 'He might bleed to death!'

It's harder, though, to accept that the media, who we assume are well informed, can perpetuate this legend. In the late 1980s it was stated on national television news that a person with haemophilia 'can bleed to death from the smallest cut.' And even as recently as 1995, a popular British television medical drama portrayed a haemophilic man who gushed blood heavily and dramatically from a nosebleed.

'Haemophilia never affects girls'

There is a widely-held conviction that girls cannot suffer from haemophilia. Whenever it is mentioned some people still respond with blank or questioning looks, but, more commonly, they say, 'Ah . . . that's the one that affects boys, isn't it?' Lack of knowledge regarding hereditary blood disorders in women stems, in part, from articles in popular publications that mislead on this point.

Von Willebrand's disease - the most common of inherited bleeding problems - crops up equally in boys and girls. And females with a very low level of Factor VIII are in the category of having mild haemophilia, yet some doctors are reluctant to acknowledge that these symptomatic carriers have actually got a blood disorder, especially one called haemophilia. Not long after haemophilia was diagnosed in Nathan, my four-year-old daughter Rachel rushed in from the garden clutching a bleeding finger. 'Mummy, help! I might be a haemophiliac,' she screamed. 'No, Rachel,' I replied firmly, 'girls can't have haemophilia.' A year later, I had to eat my words. Further blood tests confirmed that Nathan had severe haemophilia and a test on Rachel showed that she was a carrier, with only eighteen per cent of Factor VIII. In effect, she had mild haemophilia.

'No bumps or knocks'

'I suppose you have to be careful he doesn't hurt himself,' people might say on hearing your child has haemophilia. But, realistically, to do so would make any kind of family life impossible. And who wants a child wrapped in cotton wool? Possibly the hardest aspect of coping with haemophilia on a day-to-day basis is its unpredictability. Some bleeds have no obvious cause and we cannot anticipate where in the body they will occur.

'Boys should not be involved in sport in case they get injured'

If your haemophilic son takes no exercise, is never involved in any sporting activity, the result will almost certainly be a greater tendency to bleed into muscles that have no tone, into joints that are badly supported by weak muscles. Exercise will develop strong muscles to protect the joints, making them less prone to bleeds. He will grow up in a healthier body. If you encourage your child to join in some form of sport, he will feel more socially accepted, much happier than if he were left on the sidelines and you will benefit from having a better-adjusted son around.

'Mummy! I got my twenty-five metre badge for swimming today!' shouted Nathan. And I can still remember his expression. If he is unlucky enough to be injured, it's not the end of the world - his missing clotting factor is readily available.

Things people say

Comments like: 'I expect he'll grow out of it,' can be extremely difficult to cope with emotionally when, having just discovered that your child has haemophilia, you are desperately trying to accept the diagnosis. And when Nathan was young, a hospital doctor asked me, 'How long has he had haemophilia?' Clearly he didn't know much about the condition.

With such widespread confusion it is tempting to hope that the diagnosis might be wrong or that in time the disability will diminish in severity, perhaps even disappear completely. Haemophilia cannot just 'go away.' 'But he looks all right!' people exclaim, their voices echoing tones of disbelief. Your strong, normal-looking, active, happy child does not match their image of someone with this serious condition. Perhaps they expect a sudden, dramatic, visible transformation . . .

Yet haemophilia works largely unseen, deep within muscles and joints. Les was quick to point out, shortly after our son's diagnosis: 'Nathan's the same child he's always been - the only difference is that now we know about his haemophilia.'

Inform and reassure

Whatever strange things you hear, try not to be alarmed. Find out if they are true by reading about haemophilia or by asking staff at your Haemophilia Centre who will give you the facts. With information comes reassurance. Armed with knowledge you are in a good position to reassure others as well as yourself. Most importantly, inform and reassure your child from an early age. From time to time he may get odd looks from other adults. He listens in to your conversation, particularly when it concerns him . . . and probably understands more than you think. 'Why did that lady ask you if I'd had an accident?' said Nathan at the age of three.

CHAPTER FOUR

Bad Old Days

In the beginning

The Greeks were the first to write about the clotting process. The philosopher and mathematician, Pythagoras, encouraged logical study of the natural world. Empedocles applied this approach to medicine, suggesting that the body contained four 'humours': yellow bile (dry), black bile (moist), phlegm (cold) and blood (hot), all of which needed to remain in balance to ensure good health. The physician Hippocrates, observing what happened when people bled, took this theory further, stating that clotting occurred because hot blood cooled as it left the body. The Greeks described what happened when a clot formed and noticed that when a clot shrank it secreted a yellowish liquid - known today as serum.

Awareness of the existence of problems with bleeding dates back to early times. According to the Talmud, the book of Jewish law, if two boys in a Jewish family died from excessive bleeding after the religious ritual of circumcision, all subsequent boys in that family were exempt. Interestingly, the Talmud also suggested a way to staunch bleeding. 'The remedy to stop the flow of blood from a wound is 'unripe figs in vinegar'.

I remember that when I was a girl I used to drink the vinegar left over from pickling cucumbers and my mother used to say: 'That will dry your blood up!' It was as a result of William Hunter's work in the late eighteenth century that doctors began to understand more about the blood clotting process. He established a school of anatomy in London, where students applied a scientific approach to medicine. They experimented on animals and found that the action of cooling blood as it left the body delayed, rather than helped, the clotting of blood. They also deduced that plasma, the liquid part of the blood, was implicated in clotting.

The invention by Poiseville of the viscometer, an instrument which measures blood flow, stimulated doctors to make detailed studies of the action of the blood in the body. And another significant medical advance was the discovery that the proteins in blood plasma were essential to the clotting process. Some doctors in the late nineteenth century suggested that haemophilia was the result of an excess of blood in the body, while others were convinced that it was an infectious disease. Nobody knew either its cause or how to treat it.

The royal link

Haemophilia is sometimes referred to as the 'Royal Disease.' Queen Victoria and Prince Albert had nine children, five daughters and four sons. Their youngest son, Leopold, had haemophilia and two of their daughters - Alice and Beatrice -were carriers, having inherited from their mother the defective gene which causes haemophilia.

Beatrice married Prince Alexander of Battenberg, this family name being changed to the less German-sounding Mountbatten during the First World War. Out of the Mountbatten's' three boys two had haemophilia. Their daughter, Victoria, was a carrier. She married Alphonso XIII of Spain and bore him seven children. Five were sons, two were daughters. Two of the sons had haemophilia. Alice, Queen Victoria's other daughter, had seven children. One boy, Frederick, was a sufferer and two daughters - Alix and Irene - were carriers. Alix married the Russian Tsar, Nicholas II, became Empress Alexandra and the couple had a son, Alexei, born in 1904. His haemophilia was diagnosed six weeks after his birth when his umbilical cord stump, which had been a raw wound since birth, began to bleed.

A nasty fall, when he was three years old, resulted in a massive swelling on his forehead and the pressure of this bleed caused both Alexei's eyes to close.
Alexandra and the Tsar Nicholas did everything possible to protect him. They had all the trees in the royal park padded

and appointed guards to watch him while he played. They consulted the most renowned doctors of their day, but wealth and position could not change the fact that there was little that anybody could do for him when he had a bleed. Doctors advised the application of ice, splinting the affected limb and complete bed-rest. But there was no real treatment for his condition.

Finally, in desperation, Alexandra summoned the Russian monk and mystic, Rasputin, reputed to have hypnotic powers. He spent hours talking softly to the boy, which alleviated Alexei's sufferings to an astonishing degree.

Alexei was murdered at the age of fourteen by revolutionaries. Princess Irene, Alexandra's sister and Queen Victoria's granddaughter, married Henry of Prussia. Two of their three sons had haemophilia. The death of one of them, Waldemar, in 1945 marked the end of this particular network of haemophilia, which had lasted the best part of a hundred years.

First half of the twentieth century

To put it mildly, life was difficult for people with haemophilia and their parents in the first half of this century. Some doctors advised parents with a haemophilic child to move to a dry warm climate. Rural life and bathing in the sea were also considered beneficial. However, most of these parents did not get the chance to follow this advice, because over half of their affected children died before they were five. More died before adulthood and those who managed to survive were doomed to a life of inactivity: bedridden or confined to a wheelchair, their muscles wasted, their limbs deformed after years of untreated bleeds.

A 1912 Handbook for Nurses states: 'People who are known as bleeders are occasionally encountered. After the extraction of a tooth or as a result of a trivial cut, for example, such people will bleed profusely and it may be impossible to stop the haemorrhage. Probably there is some defect in the coagulating properties of the blood. Bleeders generally die early in life. There is no cure for this condition.' Such treatment as there was for people with haemophilia was at best inadequate, at worst damaging to joints and muscles.

During the next forty years matters were hardly better. Treatment for haemophilic bleeds involved raising the affected part of the body, placing ice packs around it and splinting where possible. Rest in bed followed, for days or weeks. One woman, whose father had haemophilia, said, 'I can remember he'd be in bed for a fortnight after a bleed.' Eventually, after long periods of such rest, bleeding usually stopped - but not before it had caused terrible pain and lasting damage to joints and muscles. This became a vicious cycle of bleed – prolonged rest – bleed, which led to deformed joints crippled with arthritis.

Doctors tried various ways of treating this bleeding: some suggested swallowing quantities of egg-white; others prescribed snake venom, when they could get it, for open wounds; others used elastic bandages to support muscles and lessen the flow of blood and transfusions were carried out during bad bleeds. This last form of treatment must have been particularly traumatic for children, because it was quite usual for nurses to hold them down while the doctor inserted the needle. Only rarely were parents allowed to be present.

A hospital stay for a haemophilic child meant total confinement to bed and sometimes nurses even tied them down in well-meaning attempts to prevent further injury from bumps against the cot-sides.

In the years immediately before the Second World War there were several popular medical reference books for the home, none of which offered much comfort to the parents of a haemophilic child. 'Too many cases die while still very young. Children who inherit this disease should be very carefully guarded against all accidents and operations such as tooth-pulling should only be undertaken when absolutely necessary. Daughters of haemophilic fathers should avoid marriage, as this would seem the only way to stamp out the disease.'

Breakthrough

However, shortly before the Second World War an important discovery had marked a change in the treatment of haemophilia. Research demonstrated that one of the elements in normal plasma was missing in haemophilic blood. This was AHG (anti-haemophilic globulin), now known as Factor VIII and its absence was the reason the blood-clotting process failed, causing the condition of haemophilia.

By the fifties researchers had discovered twelve clotting factors in blood and were able to separate plasma from red cells. This plasma could be kept fresh by freezing then slowly thawed and injected into a vein - and this became the standard treatment for haemophilic bleeds. However, there was the danger that, in order to maintain a high enough level of the clotting factor, too much plasma might enter the bloodstream. Such an excess could then affect the patient's heart, even cause heart failure. Doctors solved this problem when, at the beginning of the sixties, they discovered how to separate plasma into different parts. The result was cryoprecipitate - cryo meaning cold, with precipitates being the cloudy part of plasma. This product contained a lot of Factor VIII. In addition, there was some fibrinogen and factor V, other aids to clotting.

As with unseparated plasma, this cryoprecipitate was kept frozen until required. It was then thawed and injected intravenously to stop haemophilic bleeding.

But the disadvantage of cryoprecipitate, or cryo for short, was that it had to be kept frozen until needed. By 1963 Swedish doctors had concentrated Factor VIII from the rest of the blood and were injecting it into people with haemophilia to control bleeds. But even early in the sixties one medical encyclopaedia stated that a sufferer could bleed to death from a cut finger after a couple of days. With the further development of a concentrated freeze-dried form of Factor VIII, the treatment of haemophilia became much easier. This was an effective form of treatment, which could be easily transported. But it was not until the seventies that this product became widely available.

A new chapter in the history of haemophilia had begun. Uncontrolled bleeds became nightmares of the past. When home therapy was started with Factor VIII concentrate, living with haemophilia soon became less of a problem: parents could store Factor VIII in their home and inject it into their haemophilic child whenever a bleed occurred.

HIV and hepatitis

But ironically, this marvellous new lifeline also carried the potential to infect and even kill, through transmission of the virus that causes the disease AIDS from infected blood donors. This virus was first identified in May 1984. Known as HIV – Human Immunodeficiency Virus – it attacks parts of the body's immune system and can eventually break down resistance to particular types of bacteria, fungi, viruses and malignant cells. Normally when a virus, which is a tiny organism that can damage the body by invading cells, attacks us we respond by developing defensive substances called antibodies. These antibodies then attack and destroy the infection.

HIV is unusual in that it is able to survive and live alongside antibodies to it in the blood. After tests people in whom antibodies to this virus are found are termed 'HIV positive.' This means that they have been infected with and are carriers of, HIV; it does not mean they have AIDS. However, around one thousand people in the UK with haemophilia developed AIDS and died, though since 1985, when all Factor VIII has been routinely heat, chemically and detergent treated, no further cases of HIV have been identified as a result of haemophilia treatment. And twenty years on there are many HIV - infected people with haemophilia who have never developed AIDS, who seem to have some kind of inbuilt resistance.

Another serious infection transmitted through blood products was hepatitis. Virtually everyone with haemophilia who was treated with clotting factor concentrates before 1985 was infected with the hepatitis virus. Nathan was not affected, thanks to Doctor Scott, the paediatrician who treated him at West Suffolk Hospital. She was insistent that he continued to be treated with cryoprecipitate. Since this product had far fewer and known donors, unlike the more commonly used freeze-dried Factor VIII, she felt he would be less at risk from blood infections.

Three strains of hepatitis were identified, labelled A, B and C. Hepatitis A was treatable but the more serious hepatitis B and C caused liver-function impairment and sometimes death. A vaccine against hepatitis B, heat-treatment and purification of blood products were significant in reducing the risks. Ironically, it has been found that a liver transplant, sometimes necessary to save the life of a haemophilia patient with hepatitis and extensive liver damage, cures the haemophilia: sufficient Factor VIII is produced by the new liver. However, a transplant is an extremely serious and very risky procedure; not one to be undertaken in normal circumstances.

CHAPTER FIVE

Diagnosis and Modern Forms of Treatment

Out of the blue

Even when there is no known family history of the condition, severe haemophilia will almost certainly be diagnosed within the first few years. A baby who is restless and in pain from tenderness or swelling in a muscle or joint, a bad nose bleed with no apparent cause, or a cut that oozes for ages - all these are symptoms which a G.P. or hospital casualty department should recognise. Unfortunately, sometimes parents are accused of non-accidental injury - the current phrase for child battering. Haemophilia is a rare condition, child battering is considerably commoner and a doctor examining a child who has large unusual bruises is more likely to think of non-accidental injury than haemophilia. As one doctor said, 'We are not very aware of haemophilia because we don't deal with it very often.'

Increasingly, where severe bruising is present in a young child, routine blood-clotting tests are used to investigate the possibility of a blood disorder. Moderate and mild haemophilia might only be diagnosed following severe trauma, such as an operation or broken bone. Or perhaps blood tests for some other condition will show a clotting deficiency. Mild haemophilia could remain undetected for years, or even a lifetime. Equally, it can cause problems quite early in life.

Known Risk

The daughter of a man with haemophilia will be a carrier. The daughter of a woman who is a carrier has a fifty-fifty chance of being a carrier herself. DNA tests can be done on a sample of her blood to detect whether or not she is. Hopefully, a woman from a family with a history of haemophilia will have been tested for carrier status in her teens. Leaving it until she plans to or actually becomes pregnant can add an extra emotional burden. Decision-making about becoming a parent of a possibly affected child is a very sensitive area. If a woman is a carrier or has a partner with haemophilia they can obtain free genetic counselling and antenatal tests. Specially trained staff will handle all the issues involved with sensitivity. Your local Haemophilia Centre or the Haemophilia Society will advise you where such facilities are available.

Testing for haemophilia antenatally used to be a hazardous process and so was only undertaken when a termination was an agreed possibility. Chorionic villus sampling, which involves taking cells from the baby's side of the placenta in early pregnancy and subjecting the cells to DNA analysis, is now the usual method of testing for haemophilia. The result is almost completely reliable; it does, however, carry a small but significant risk of miscarriage. Those who are deterred by any risk to their pregnancy can instead opt for ultrasonic scanning, which can be carried out any time after sixteen weeks. This is a safe, non-invasive procedure, which reveals the sex of the baby and allows, if the foetus is male, emotional and mental preparation for the fifty-fifty chance of haemophilia in the baby.

Treatment

When deciding on treatment, the doctor takes account of both the size and seriousness of the bleed, the severity of the haemophilia and the weight of the child. This information determines the amount of medication necessary. If a child is severely affected, the normal treatment is with recombinant Factor VIII, a safer alternative to the conventional product in that it is not produced from human plasma, which carries the risk of viral infections. One problem is the enormous cost of the product. Another is the high demand for it.

A minor bleed in a person with mild or moderate haemophilia or Von Willebrand's Disease may be treated with injections of desmopressin - a synthetic substance similar to a hormone produced by the pituitary gland in the brain. Early treatment is essential to maintain healthy joints and muscles. The amount of rest needed after a bleed is determined by the severity of the pain. However, the sooner a child is mobilised, the better. After a muscle or joint bleed, some physiotherapy may increase mobility and speed up the body's ability to disperse any dried blood left behind when a bleed is over. The physiotherapist designs a plan of treatment for each person to suit their particular problem. Exercise and physiotherapy in a heated pool and ultra-sound treatment might be included in such a plan. For example, with Nathan they used what looked like a small, slender microphone under water to disperse the debris of a bleed into a finger joint. And he watched, fascinated.

Pain control

Early treatment of a bleed is the first and most important step in managing pain; the sooner treatment is given, the less the pain. Delay in treatment increases the likelihood of damage to joints and muscles as well as greater pain. Anaesthetic creams, applied to the skin before an injection, make the treatment procedure virtually painless. These can be prescribed by your doctor. Any pain from a bleed needs to be treated early and regularly with a moderately strong painkiller – there are several suitable preparations; however, *never* use one containing any form of aspirin, since this thins the blood and prolongs bleeding. If a stronger painkiller is required, consult your doctor. Fortunately, severe pain is rarely a problem nowadays. Drugs are not the only way to control pain. After a bleed into a muscle or joint, crushed ice placed in a wet towel and packed around the affected part for ten minutes may help to decrease the swelling and bring relief. You can even use a bag of frozen peas! (They can safely be refrozen afterwards.) And warmth can sometimes help. Immerse the joint or muscle in a large bowl of warm water. If this cannot be done, ten minutes of a wrapped hot-water bottle on the affected part of the body can alleviate the pain.

Cold and heat methods can be alternated. Both improve blood supply to the painful part and this speeds up the healing process. A cold compression wrap is a useful short-term aid. This can be purchased from larger chemists. It is a specially impregnated bandage that cools, compresses and supports the affected area. It is reusable and is stored in the freezer. Gentle exercise when a bleed has stopped usually helps to restore mobility as well as reducing possible residual pain.

Prophylaxis

When Nathan was little, it was usual to treat bleeds with injections as and when they occurred. Only occasionally was prophylaxis (i.e. preventative treatment) advised. When he had a spate of recurrent bleeds into his left ankle at the age of eight, I was advised to give him three injections a week to allow him normal mobility. This lasted for about three months. It was necessary not to always use the same vein because of the risk of damage from over-use and to use firm pressure for several minutes afterwards with cotton wool at the injection site in order to preserve the veins.

The trend now is to give regular, ongoing treatment to severely affected children two to three times a week, until the child has stopped growing to prevent rather than treat joint damage. This is only commenced when the child has had a couple of bleeds and seems likely to run into recurrent problems. The veins in very young children are hard to locate because of their size so this is achieved by implanting a small device called a Portacath into a large vein under the skin of the chest wall or under the armpit. This has a small entry port to allow for easy injecting, so that parents can inject their child without difficulty. The haematologist at your Haemophilia Centre will advise you if or when this is necessary and staff will give you plenty of training and support. Some parents (and children) prefer this method. It does not inhibit normal activity and the use of an anaesthetic cream on the skin shortly before an injection means there is little or no pain involved.

However, there is the ever-present danger of complacency: if bleeds are not occurring it is very important for your child to know that they still have the condition, that prophylaxis does not give complete immunity from bleeds. The child does not become Superman, with the ability to jump off a garage roof without damage! Nothing in life is risk-free; there is always a risk of infection or thrombosis from the use of a Portacath. Regular inspection by the staff at your Haemophilia Centre will ensure that if this occurs it is dealt with promptly. When a child's veins are more prominent parents may prefer to have the Portacath removed (ideally by the age of six) and to inject directly into a vein in an arm or hand. Anaesthetic creams make this a fairly painless process.

'Thanks to modern methods of treatment,' Nathan's haematologist, Doctor Adelman says, 'We no longer see the haemophilia patient with the typical bent walk and chronic joint deformities.' A great advantage of prophylactic treatment over treatment 'on demand' (i.e. when bleeds occur) is the prevention of spontaneous bleeding by increasing the Factor VIII level in the blood to that of mild haemophilia.

When to treat

Although emergency dashes to hospital are rare for the person with haemophilia, certain bleeds need very prompt treatment over and above the need for Factor VIII – for instance deep cuts, suspected broken bones, blows to the head. Even at night, a haematologist is on call and should be consulted immediately for advice. Cuts requiring stitches can be temporarily stopped from bleeding with firm pressure until medical attention is given. There are other reasons to seek medical advice such as an unusually severe headache, an unexplainable pain in any part of the body, any obvious swelling, damage to the face, mouth, eyes or tongue (Small tongue bites may stop of their own accord after oozing for longer than usual: sucking an ice-cube or ice lollipop might be helpful). Where a bleed has started in a joint or muscle it needs to be treated before it becomes too swollen and painful. Those affected gradually learn to recognise when a bleed is beginning. Parents and doctors are often guided by this feeling, which can precede any visible signs.

Early and adequate replacement of the missing clotting factor is extremely important, as it lessens considerably the chance of any long-term damage to joints and muscles. The fibres, thread-like structure in muscles, are gradually destroyed if a muscle bleed is left too long untreated. And useless muscles cannot support joints. The golden rule is to give treatment whenever you suspect a bleed. If in doubt, treat. Never just ignore it in the hope that it will 'go away.' It rarely does without leaving some damage in its wake. If you need any advice, help is just a phone call away.

Home therapy

An important advance in the management of haemophilia was the introduction of home treatment in the mid-1970s. The main advantages of home therapy over other ways of dealing with haemophilia are early replacement of the clotting factor and a greater degree of personal control over the condition. And familiar surroundings can make everyone feel more relaxed. The whole experience is less disruptive of family life.

However, before home therapy can start parents must actually want to do it. If a Portacath has been implanted, home treatment can begin early in a child's life at around a year to eighteen months after a course of training.

Once the decision is made to treat at home, staff at your Centre will give all necessary advice for storage of the Factor VIII and its preparation. The Factor is kept in the fridge. There needs to be an area of a room where treatment can be hygienically prepared with a 'sharps bin' at hand for the disposal of needles and syringes. Treatment packs are delivered to the patient's home or workplace on average every two months. They contain everything needed for injections: bottles of Factor VIII, sterile distilled water used to reconstitute it, needles, syringes, skin cleansers, cotton wool...

Parents keep a written record of each treatment. All home treatment is monitored by staff at the Haemophilia Centre who keep a record of everything issued to patients. In time your child will begin self-infusion. This may be at any time from the age of ten to the teens. This process is made easier if you encourage him to help in the treatment procedures from a very early age, explaining each step and the need for hygiene in terms appropriate to his age. And explaining the reasons for regular injections broadens understanding about his condition.

The haemophilia staff will give friendly advice and support whenever you need it. Sister Brenda's help was invaluable when I injected Nathan at home. And nowadays Nathan rings Ally, Brenda's successor in Lincoln, whenever he needs to.

Operations

Except in an emergency, if an operation is necessary the patient needs to go into hospital at least twenty-four hours beforehand. Before any surgical procedure, no matter how small, a test must be carried out to ensure that there are no antibodies to Factor VIII. Doctors calculate the required dose of clotting factor and it is given before surgery and for several days afterwards to keep the clotting level as near normal as possible until the wound from the operation has healed. So any surgical procedure can be carried out without excessive bleeding. The entire procedure is probably as safe for a person with haemophilia as for any other patient.

In an emergency operation, this same process is speeded up to meet the patient's clotting needs throughout and following the operation.

Risk factors from treatment

There is a theoretical risk of the transmission of vCJD (variant Creutzfeldt-Jacob Disease) from products using human or animal-derived protein additives. But in March 2004 ADVATE was launched in the UK. This is a new treatment product for haemophilia and is the only Factor VIII made without the use of such proteins at any stage during its manufacture. At the time of writing, another product is under clinical trials.

In time, all children newly diagnosed will be treated with these third generation products. And plasma-derived products, still currently used for people with haemophilia over forty-one on account of the high cost of recombinant Factor, are now all imported (mainly from the USA) in an attempt to avoid any risk of CJD contamination.

Inhibitors

Inhibitors are a major problem in a small number of people with haemophilia. Although many develop inhibitors when they first start regular treatment, most disappear of their own accord. Factor VIII is a foreign protein to someone with severe haemophilia and the body is not accustomed to having it in the blood in high quantity. If you inject a substance that the body perceives as foreign, it can produce antibodies. These are called inhibitors. They inhibit, or prevent, the Factor VIII from working effectively in the clotting process by attaching themselves to the Factor VIII molecules as they enter the blood and destroying them, which is an obvious problem; the usual doses of Factor VIII no longer work because the patient has become immune.

A blood test can determine if a person has developed an inhibitor. So what can be done for someone with inhibitors who needs treatment? One way is to continue regular treatment with higher than normal amounts until the body becomes tolerant of Factor VIII and the antibody level drops. Another is to treat bleeds with a product such as Novoseven, which is able to bypass the need for Factor VIII, is unaffected by inhibitors and has been developed for this purpose.

For all children undergoing immune-tolerance treatment to eradicate inhibitors a Portacath is a necessity because it reduces the number of injections into a vein. Because of the complexities of dealing with inhibitors, the treatment is always closely monitored by your Comprehensive Care Centre.

CHAPTER SIX

Day To Day

Infancy

An unborn child with haemophilia is well protected inside the amniotic sac (the bag of waters) in its mother's womb. There is the same chance of normal pregnancy for this baby as for any other and birth presents no increased danger. If a diagnosis is reached prenatally, or soon after birth, parents will feel anxious about the new arrival, especially if the baby is their first born.

Many of us are unsure, first time around, about handling our seemingly fragile newborn infant. My first baby, Simon, was born small for dates and weighed little more than two bags of sugar. And to this day I can remember feeling how frightened I was of dropping him and being left with the empty shawl! Even holding him tightly seemed dangerous. A diagnosis of haemophilia can intensify that uncertainty. It is not only perfectly safe for parents, relatives and friends to pick up, to cuddle the haemophilic baby in the usual way... it is essential.

A tiny baby senses, soaks up its mother's feelings. Her tone of voice, her touch will transmit love, happiness, enjoyment - or fear, tension, sadness. Emotional development begins here. So love your baby, enjoy each milestone and encourage others to do the same. There is something very special about that first smile, that first roll over, the first gurgle, sitting up, standing up. Your baby is no more likely to come to harm than any other baby of this age.

And vaccinations are as important for the haemophilic baby as for others. They should be given intravenously (into a vein) or subcutaneously (under the skin), rather than into the muscle, which could cause a bleed. Apply firm pressure for about five minutes afterwards. Use normal baby equipment: carrycot, rocking cradle, baby bouncer, playpen, baby walker, highchair and cot. Special measures such as padding the furniture or cot are unnecessary.

Once your baby begins to crawl take the same sort of sensible safety precautions you would for all mini-explorers - stair-gates, fireguard, cooker guard, no sharp-edged toys, car safety seat... Treat your child no differently from other children. Encourage play with others - vital for healthy, normal physical and emotional development. Resist the natural urge to over-protect your child.

Accepting the diagnosis

If there is no known family history it is normal to experience numbness on first learning that your child has haemophilia. This natural reaction is nature's way of protecting us from the full impact of sudden, enormous shock. The diagnosis is too much to take in straight away. You may block it out; you may pretend that nothing has happened, simply carry on, robot-like, with normal functions and familiar routine.

Just one look at your bright, beautiful child is enough to belie the words: 'Your child has haemophilia.' And the shocked responses to the news of relatives and friends emphasise your denial of what has happened. 'Perhaps they've got it wrong,' they say and 'Maybe it's not as bad as they think.' They, too, cannot believe the diagnosis at first.

You also hope that the doctors are mistaken. You don't want to accept the truth because it's too painful. But once the numbness wears off and you begin to hurt, you need to express these painful feelings of grief, anger, guilt, inadequacy, fear. Give yourself the opportunity to cry, rage, grieve and work through the emotions on your own and with sympathetic listeners who understand the terrible pain. Only then can you begin to fully believe and accept that your child has a blood disorder that can be easily treated if not yet cured and start to resume a full, happy family life.

When you are ready to believe that your child has haemophilia, look at the beautiful person that you played a part in creating, of whom you are so proud. Notice those smiles, listen to the happy laughter and watch for the loving looks that are so rewarding. Love will help to soothe your pain. Don't confuse the child with the condition. The diagnosis has not changed your child, who is still the same lovable person you have always known. Early on we stopped labelling Nathan a 'haemophiliac', regarding him instead as our delightful little son who happened to have a condition called haemophilia.

You will learn not only to cope but to cope well, even though you may not, at first, see how. This book is testimony to the fact that it is perfectly possible to progress from being frightened, over-protective and unhappy, to the point where haemophilia recedes into the background, with relationships strengthened along the way. Once you begin to accept your child's haemophilia you have the energy and will power to find out more about it, to enlighten others about it and to draw on inner resources to cope.

You can do nothing to change the fact of haemophilia, but you can do much to change your own and others' attitudes towards it.

One day at a time

'If only I hadn't said. . .' I have learnt the hard way how easy it is to acquire the 'If only . . .' mentality - an utterly pointless way of thinking. No amount of fretting over the past makes any difference; we cannot undo what has already happened.

'What will happen if . . .?' Worrying about tomorrow, next week, next year will not change the future. What it will do though is drain our resources, leave us feeling weak, disheartened and unhappy.

Obviously it is necessary to give some thought to the future - booking holidays, taking out insurance, making appointments - but being anxious about something that may or may not happen is an absolute waste of time. Far better to use all our energy for 'here and now.' And it is amazing how many things, often little things, can give pleasure even during a difficult day- your child's laughter, a beautiful flower, a loving touch - all easily missed if your thoughts are far away in the past or the future. There were times when Nathan's beautiful smile helped put everything in perspective for me.

When Nathan's haemophilia was diagnosed all my thoughts and fears centred on the future. I was fraught with worry over his safety. Lots of 'what ifs' crowded my mind, making me unbearably anxious, tense and depressed.

In desperation I tried limiting my concerns to one day - today - to live in 'day-tight compartments'. It was like taking off several unnecessary layers of heavy clothing. My mind felt lighter, my concentration improved and it was easier to cope. If you have just found out about your child's haemophilia, try not to think about what might have been or what might be, only what is - today. Occupying yourself and keeping busy leave no time for anxiety.

Spending time with your child talking, reading, singing, playing games... you get to know each other better and your relationship improves. 'I like it when we come to hospital,' said Nathan to me one day, 'because then we can talk to each other.'

Instead of dwelling on the possibility of future bleeds, think about this Jewish saying: 'Only one kind of worry is proper, to worry because you worry so much.'

Know your enemy

Your worries will often disappear in the light of what you know. Once you have accepted your child's haemophilia, you can think more clearly but may still find it frightening. The unknown is much more frightening than the known. And mistakes and misconceptions - our own and others - fuel the fear. So find out everything you can about haemophilia - read about it and talk with people who know a lot about the condition such as the doctor at your Centre, who treats haemophilia every day.

It's a good idea to write down your questions before you get there. It can be very annoying to remember all the questions you wanted to ask when you have left the hospital! And if you do not understand the answers ask again: in common with most professionals, doctors have a jargon of their own. When you get home write down the facts so that you can refer to them another day. Reminding yourself of what you already know gives you confidence: real facts are never as frightening as imagined ones. And because you now have some idea of what you are up against, you are far better equipped to cope with haemophilia. You feel less inadequate, less helpless, more in control.

Over Protection

When haemophilia is first diagnosed it is tempting to try to give total protection to prevent further bleeds. You may aim to provide an ultra-safe environment that will shield your toddler from any possible harm. But are you going to tell your him that running, jumping, hopping, skipping, climbing ... all the recently acquired skills, practised daily with confidence and pride, are forbidden from now on? Just as you cannot stop a butterfly in flight without damage, you cannot permanently stop your child from living life to the full without inflicting lasting harm. To do so would transform any lively, healthy, well-adjusted child into a weak, unhappy one afraid to venture out. The child, sensing your fear, would cling to you for protection. And how much healthier it was to have Nathan scrambling up his climbing frame into his 'den' than sitting watching television.

However, taking a few sensible precautions that are not extreme will make you feel more in control - buy round-edged furniture and toys, throw out the rusty lawn mower, repair cracks in the garden path... Your toddler needs to experience life and living to the full by playing, testing, exploring, enjoying the environment and making friends. Praising his achievements, big or small, will develop his confidence.

The unpredictability of severe haemophilia can mean a bleed at rest or play, so whatever the measures you take you can never guarantee a bleed-free existence. But by allowing your toddler to live normally you will promote normal healthy development - mentally, emotionally and physically.

Supervise all activity in the same way you would with any other small child and join in with some. But avoid the temptation to issue a stream of 'Don'ts!'
Of course you are always conscious of haemophilia, but do not let it cloud your vision. First and foremost, see your child as a normal child . . . who just happens to have haemophilia.

After a bleed

Days, sometimes weeks, of boredom spent in bed recovering from a bleed, belong to the past. Today, prophylaxis has made life easier; and if your child does have a bleed, factor replacement soon after it has started means restriction for only short periods, if at all. After treatment for an acute bleed into a muscle or joint, a careful balance is needed. Too much rest will result in wasted muscles, unstable joints, more bleeds. Too little will not allow for full recovery and bleeding may start again.

A little common sense goes a long way. In the case of a small tongue bleed, for instance, avoiding giving hard foods like toast or biscuits for a few days gives it a good chance to heal fully. If your young child needs to spend a day or so in hospital try to stay with him. Most hospitals have a room where parents can sleep. Bring in a favourite toy or comforter to cuddle. Familiar items are important at this time.

If you cannot stay overnight, leave something like your glove, then it will be obvious that you have to return.

Answer all his questions simply and honestly. Use this brief time to build a stronger relationship with your child. Talk, read, sing, play board games together. 'If life hands you a lemon, make lemonade.'

Any over-reaction is counter-productive. A child needs the company of other children, needs some of the rough and tumble of normal childhood. Nathan was a very active child who enjoyed playing boisterously with his family and friends. If there are no brothers or sisters, take your child to a playgroup, visit friends with young children. Invite friends round. Provided everyone involved understands the condition and knows your contact number if the need arises, you can safely leave your child with friends. Get a babysitter; enjoy an evening out with your partner. Dad is as important in a child's life as Mum. It is healthy for them to romp around in the same way as they would if the child did not have haemophilia. The same 'do's and don'ts' apply as for any other child -though too many will lead to frustration for the pair of you! It's fine to play with toys, ride pedal cars, tricycles... Go swimming, to the park, to the seaside. Do all the normal things you would with any child of this age. Enjoy your young child. Those early years fly fast.

Starting school

Most people with haemophilia go to normal schools. Talk with your child about the sort of things he will do each day at school.

Some anxiety is natural as he disappears into the classroom on his first day, as well as the usual apprehensions that any mother experiences when her child first starts school. In addition, your mind might buzz with questions like, 'What if another child pushes him over in the playground?', 'How will others react if he hurts himself?'

There are ways to make starting school easier.

Well before the beginning of the school term make an appointment to talk to the head teacher and the class teacher. Give them information about your child's condition. The Haemophilia Society provides a booklet, *Haemophilia in the Classroom*. Discuss the sort of activities that your child can join in - the more the better. Explain the need for your child to be treated as normally as possible. The teacher's attitude will affect the child's attitude to school. It will also influence other children's attitudes. Ask that no allowance be made for bad behaviour or poor quality work. Haemophilia is no excuse for either. Discuss any realistic precautions you feel are necessary to guard against bleeds.

Ensure staff know how to contact you at any time. Explain: -

a) What prophylactic treatment means.

b) Small cuts or grazes only need treating in the usual way – cleansed and a plaster applied. Perhaps two, if blood oozes through the first.

c) A person with haemophilia bleeds no faster than anybody else, although the blood cannot clot in the normal way. Most bleeds are into joints and muscles.

d) There is no need for panic. From the onset of a bleed to its full development is usually a gradual process.

e) Any pain, with or without swelling in a muscle or joint, probably needs treatment and may or may not be warm to the touch.

f) Heavy or persistent external bleeding can be stopped with pressure until treatment is available. The usual first aid measures work just the same for the person with haemophilia as for anyone else.

g) You need to be notified immediately in the event of any cause for concern, such as a blow on the head or complaint of severe pain.

Importance of exercise

Regular exercise is important for everyone, including those with haemophilia. It not only makes us look and feel healthier, it also relieves stress, stimulates good blood circulation and promotes strong muscle tone. And powerful muscles protect joints. Unexercised muscles become weak, flabby and, in the person with haemophilia, more subject to bleeds. If gentle exercise is not begun soon after a muscle bleed, the muscle contracts, affecting a joint which then fails to work properly. A physiotherapist can recommend exercises to help restore full mobility after a bleed, exercises for strengthening particular muscles.

Encourage your child to discover an enjoyable sport, remembering that any limitations are far better learnt than imposed. Swimming is a particularly suitable activity for people with haemophilia because it uses every muscle and can even be resumed shortly after a bleed since little weight bearing is involved. Nathan was able to take part in his school's swimming gala despite a recent bleed into a big toe joint. It is important when resting one part of the body after a bleed that the whole body does not fall into disuse.

Participation in more competitive sports is to be encouraged. Volleyball, table tennis, badminton, athletics can, on occasion, result in injury for anyone, with or without haemophilia. Banning all sport for your child will cause more problems than it solves. You may provoke feelings of isolation, unhappiness, resentment... Forbid reasonable risk taking and you might be defied. Worse still, it may lead to unacceptable risks. It is normal for people with haemophilia to feel the need to prove themselves, to demonstrate their ability to fit in with a peer group. Recognising and accepting these feelings helps you to boost self esteem and confidence - invaluable aids for the future.

Naturally the correct equipment should be worn for the sport. For example, shin pads when playing soccer and shock-absorbing soles inside jogging shoes. If bleeds occur they can usually be treated quite quickly with easily transportable Factor VIII. Nathan's paediatrician frequently talked about her experiences with people with haemophilia in the Canadian Rockies. They were keen to pursue their sport of canoeing, so accepted the inevitable injections. A few sports, however, are inadvisable. Any direct body contact sport such as rugby, boxing, wrestling and karate is best avoided.

Diet

It is important to keep weight at a normal level in order to avoid the problem of strain on joints and muscles and the difficulty of finding a vein in someone who is obese. A healthy diet, with plenty of fruit and vegetables rather than junk food, combined with regular exercise, is essential for a child with haemophilia (or for anyone else, for that matter!).

Don't panic!

How your child behaves when a bleed occurs will very much depend on how you react. Any panic will not only show in your eyes, it will also be evident in a raised voice, agitated movements and be felt in trembling hands. Whatever happens, try to breathe slowly, deeply, steadily and remain outwardly calm for your child's sake.

If you stay in control during a crisis you convey the message that this situation is controllable. Which it usually is, even if at first it appears otherwise. One night, when Nathan was seven, he woke me complaining that one of his eyes would not open - the eyelids had stuck together. Half asleep I followed him through the semi-darkness into the bathroom to wash his face. 'What's this?' he said, fingering his face. I switched on the light and was horrified to see that Nathan's eye was covered in blood. Dried blood also covered his face, hands and most of his pyjama top. Our voices woke Les, who came to investigate. 'I'll call an ambulance,' he said.

'No, wait!' I said, 'let's see where it's coming from first.'

'It's blood, Mummy!' Nathan's voice rose in alarm as he looked at his hands, saw my expression and heard the fear in his daddy's voice. Unless we at least appeared to be coping, it was clear that Nathan was likely to lose control. He might scream and that would wake the other children, who could also panic. I lifted him into the bath and forced myself to speak quietly, comfortingly. Nathan, who was not in any pain, visibly relaxed. I washed away the dried blood and discovered the source -blood was trickling from one of his nostrils. 'It's only a nosebleed, no need to phone,' I said.

Normal first aid measures stopped the small flow that had made such a big mess. We cleaned Nathan up, changed the bedclothes and tucked him in. Nathan had watched my reactions throughout. 'I'm glad it was just a nose bleed,' he said sleepily as I kissed him.

Familiarity diminishes fear

Anyone who lives constantly with a condition, any condition, eventually becomes more or less accustomed to it. Nasty bruises, swollen joints, painful muscles, oozing cuts, the different ways in which haemophilia can manifest itself, become familiar signs in time. You find better ways of organising any visits to hospital, like keeping a bag packed with toys and other essentials for the unexpected trip. You learn to expect the unexpected. You find ways to deal with pain, ways to comfort your child. Understanding the nature of haemophilia, you begin to feel some degree of control over it. Both you and he begin to recognise when a bleed has occurred. You learn to trust instinct and treat bleeds at an early stage. The routine of treatment has a familiar pattern.

CHAPTER SEVEN

A Helping Hand

Haemophilia Centres

Haemophilia Centres were established over forty years ago. By working together they were able to ensure nationally accepted standards of diagnosis and treatment of haemophilia. They could also collate and pool information about the condition. After our family moved to Lincolnshire we were grateful for the friendliness and expertise of staff at Lincoln County Hospital's well-run Haemophilia Centre. Every Centre has a Director, a doctor who is responsible for ensuring daily, round-the-clock, readily available treatment for haemophilic bleeds and regular reviews for its patients. A specially trained haemophilia nursing sister can support, help, advise and befriend you. Laboratory staff diagnose blood disorders, monitor patients' treatment and perform tests on treatment products and patients' blood, to detect any detrimental changes in either.

Comprehensive Care Centres

There are twenty-six Comprehensive Care Centres in the UK at the time of writing, some of them treating children and adults, others being specifically for children who then transfer to a nearby adult centre. The age of the changeover varies with the centre, the youngest being sixteen years, the eldest eighteen.

As well as providing the normal facilities of a haemophilia centre, a comprehensive care centre also provides a specialist consultant service for all procedures beyond the scope of the smaller units, which will refer patients to them when necessary. They also act as training centres and co-ordinate research programmes and clinical trials. Additionally, there is often a senior nurse who works in the community, giving home treatment and advice where needed.

The GP and the local hospital

Everyone who has haemophilia must be registered with a general practitioner who will be kept informed of any treatment given and other relevant details. The GP needs to know such information when consulted about common infections and illnesses and in case of an emergency. If you live some way from a Haemophilia Centre a well-informed local doctor can be enormously helpful in deciding whether or not a trip to hospital is necessary. Some are even willing to inject haemophilic patients, who live some distance from the nearest hospital. They keep a ready supply of Factor VIII refrigerated in their surgery.

In an unfamiliar area telephone the haematologist at the local District Hospital to explain your situation. In this way a haemophilic bleed can be treated quickly, thus avoiding long delays and unnecessary X-rays in the Casualty Department. If an ambulance is needed to take someone with haemophilia to hospital the crew must be informed of the severity of a particular bleed. If the situation is urgent, a fast response is vital.

Support Groups

The World Federation of Hemophilia (American spelling of haemophilia) was founded in 1963 by Frank Schnabel, who was himself severely affected. It incorporates many national Haemophilia Societies and provides an essential service by working with other worldwide organisations, such as the Red Cross, to help people with haemophilia and their families in the Third World. Often there is a complete lack of resources for the diagnosis and treatment of blood disorders in these countries, since malnutrition inevitably takes priority over haemophilia. The W.F.H. also meets regularly with its own member groups and other international organisations concerned with disability, to discuss ways of improving life for people with haemophilia.

The Haemophilia Society

The W.F.H. numbered the United Kingdom-based Haemophilia Society, established in 1950, among its first members. Back in the 1930s a number of patients with haemophilia felt the need to meet, on a regular basis, at a London hospital. These meetings led to the foundation of The Haemophilia Society, whose membership has since been extended to include relatives of people with haemophilia and other blood disorders and anyone interested in the condition. It is an important organisation, which gives help in many ways as I have found from personal experience.

The Society campaigns vigorously for the rights of people with haemophilia including those affected by viruses from blood products and makes representations to Government on their behalf. It works hard too to secure the best possible treatment for blood disorders and gives up-to-date information about all new developments to its members and health care professionals. Members receive helpful literature, a regular news update, called HQ and a great deal of other assistance in many areas of life - travel, employment and benefits...

They provide details of a scheme to provide a free pager for parents of children under sixteen. In addition, they run heavily subsidised holidays for youngsters aged eight to thirteen with haemophilia and related blood disorders as well as their brothers and sisters. When Nathan was eight he greatly enjoyed one such holiday in Wales which included rock-climbing and abseiling, giving him his first taste of independence. Full supervision and medical care were part of the package.

Local support groups

The Haemophilia Society or your local centre can put you in contact with your nearest support group. It can help to talk to others who have experience of what you are going through. 'I never realised that others felt like me . . .' Parents can easily feel isolated with their worries and fears about a newly diagnosed haemophilic child. The listening ears and empathy of others who understand haemophilia-related problems may be just what they need to be better able to cope with their situation.

Groups have a committee whose members are responsible for financial and general management. Some also run a twenty-four hour telephone service and pay supportive visits to families. By discussing problems with their Centre Director they can, if necessary, often bring about improvements in standards of treatment. Members of the group meet regularly for social and fund-raising events. And Nathan and our other children greatly enjoyed activities organised by our local group, such as Christmas parties, theme park outings and trips to the seaside.

Useful Equipment

A very soft toothbrush is a small, but important item. Some of the bacteria that develop in any plaque that remains on teeth cause tooth decay, others cause gum disease. And gum disease causes bleeding. By brushing twice daily with a really soft brush your child can clean teeth very close to the gums. This should ensure complete removal of plaque. Ankle bleeds in your active haemophilic child can sometimes be a problem. 'The ankle joint is the second commonest site of bleeding in the under 12 age group,' wrote Joyce Lovering in the Haemophilia Society Bulletin; the knee being commonest.

Try giving your child supportive boots to wear, they may help. You can buy high-sided trainers for young children and Doctor Martin or similar boots for older boys. Nathan was very comfortable in his high-sided trainers and keen to wear them.

If an injury has occurred, protection is also required sometimes for elbows and knees, as well as ankles. Foam padding can be stuck inside an appropriate length of tubular stretch stocking, which can be prescribed by your doctor. Worn during the daytime, unseen under trousers or shirt, this can help to prevent further bleeds. Or you can buy it ready-made: 'Tubipad' is available from the larger chemists that sell surgical appliances as well as from Internet suppliers.

Another aid that you can buy in sports shops are Sorbothane insoles to put inside shoes. Designed primarily for joggers they are very soft and reduce the impact of everyday movements on ankles and knees. Crutches and wheelchairs can be useful short-term aids. The chair may have an elevated footrest attachment, which provides extra support and comfort for a painful lower limb. My GP prescribed a wheelchair during a series of ankle bleeds when Nathan was five. It allowed him to continue attending school and was useful when taking him for treatment after an ankle bleed.

To avoid weakening muscles it is important only to use such aids for the minimum time necessary. Your local Social Services Department also has an Occupational Therapist, who will be happy to visit you to assess your child's needs with a view to loaning other useful equipment.

A MedicAlert identity bracelet or neck pendant, worn particularly when your child spends any time away from you, contains all necessary information about his particular condition. Your local centre will provide a green card with the nature of the blood disorder, the factor level and a contact phone number. Knowing that your haemophilic child is protected in this way is reassuring. An ambulance crew would look for such identification and valuable time could be saved on arrival at hospital.

Department of Health and Social Security entitlements

Once your haemophilic child is three months old you may be entitled to claim Disability Allowance. And if he is three or over and prone to bleeds into lower limbs, you could be entitled to Mobility Component Disability Allowance. The

Haemophilia Society will keep you up-to-date regarding benefits for people with haemophilia.

Back-up support in education

An ancillary helper in school is usually only provided if your child has inhibitors as well as severe haemophilia. If this is the case ask your Health Visitor about the legal process of Statementing. As it can take eighteen months to two years to complete the procedure, it is best started when your child is three years old. Once the Health Visitor has set the wheels in motion, an educational advisor, doctor, educational psychologist and nurse or your Health Visitor will assess whether or not special supervision is necessary. Your own opinions and feelings will be taken into account and, when a decision is reached, you will receive copies of the assessments.

Family Support

You are not alone! Doctors, nursing staff, physiotherapists, teachers, social workers and many local groups and organisations exist to help you. But unless you speak up they may not know that you need them. The Haemophilia Society is interested too in your family and offers support, advice and information. If you need help - ask.

CHAPTER EIGHT

Proper Perspective

The person or the disability?

'As you go through life make this your goal, Keep your eye upon the doughnut and not upon the hole.' (Doughnut Cafe, Melbourne)

'Everyone treats me like a baby when I'm in a wheelchair,' Nathan said crossly.

Someone had just stopped us to ask me what was wrong with my son and had then bent down to speak to him in the special voice some people use when talking to babies, the mentally handicapped or someone in a wheelchair. So it was hardly surprising that my child who just the day before had been treated as a normal eight-year-old when he was walking, running and jumping, would feel confused and angry when people's attitude towards him changed dramatically the moment he was confined to a wheelchair.

He now had two problems to face - recovery after a bad ankle bleed and the condescension of others. The sight of anybody in a wheelchair often has a profound effect on people: it provokes curiosity and can arouse feelings of pity. And when the occupant is a child those feelings are magnified. People may stare or move away pretending to have seen nothing. They often assume that the inability to walk is coupled with an incapacity for coherent speech or thought and talk only to the person pushing the wheelchair.

When people talk or write about a disability they often fail to do more than make passing reference to the sufferer. Yet everyone is a person with a unique personality; nothing should ever detract from that, it is always possible to see the real person, however severe a disability. And often that person is a vibrant, interesting human being, willing to interact with others given half a chance.

I once read an article about a young severely haemophilic child. There was a reasonable amount of information about haemophilia and the problems his parents have to cope with, but information about the boy himself was scant and limited to age, place in family.... I could not even begin to imagine what sort of child he was, not even a picture was included. So I was left with a good clinical view of the condition and regrets that the writer had concentrated on the missing clotting factor, while missing the human factor.

Looking at Nathan I am often deeply moved by his beauty and by the love, warmth, sensitivity, intelligence and zest for life that shines in those dark brown eyes. His haemophilia is of secondary importance.

What is 'normal'?

The dictionary describes it as according to rule, not deviating from the standard, ordinary, well-adjusted, functioning regularly. Defined in these terms - is anybody really normal? Once we get to know a disabled person, the handicap no longer looms large but fades into the background where it belongs. But if the disability is not immediately obvious, as in haemophilia, the person is regarded and treated as normal until the condition is revealed, when others may react with fear, shock, perhaps disbelief because they cannot see the disability.

Attitudes may then change and it is fear of this that causes some people with haemophilia to keep the condition secret. One man said, 'I try not to let people know that I have haemophilia, because when they know they don't treat me normally: they pity me.' A person with haemophilia is an absolutely normal person - apart from having a blood disorder.

Boundaries

The haemophilic child has all the same basic needs of any child for food, love, protection, discipline... Carefully thought out discipline makes a child feel wanted, protected and loved. It is proof that the adults in the child's life care enough to provide clear limits within which it is safe to express feelings and develop potential.

Inflexibility, however, is harmful and produces negative responses: repression, shyness, rebellion, lack of confidence, phobias. And attempts to control behaviour with threats of injections or visits to hospital destroy trust and instil fear of treatment. As does punishing your child for not telling you sooner about a bleed. Little or inconsistent discipline is also damaging because it creates feelings of confusion, unhappiness, insecurity, self-centredness and a person who may ultimately be unable to relate closely and lovingly to anyone. A spoilt haemophilic child will grow up with two disabilities instead of one. We cannot take away a physical problem, but we can guard against adding an emotional one. A well-disciplined child learns self-discipline and self-responsibility; learns to cope with crises, with haemophilia and grows up in greater safety.

Parents spoil a child with a disability for various reasons - love, guilt and the desire to compensate. Sadly, where parents give whatever is requested and allow anti-social, unacceptable behaviour, they convey the fallacy that the world exists solely for that child's benefit. The result - a person whom nobody likes.

Haemophilia as a weapon

Andrew, a bright seven-year old, had severe haemophilia. He didn't like his new school and few people liked him. His teacher said, 'Andrew has not settled in well here. When he started he told other children in the playground that they were not allowed to hit him because of his haemophilia. But he seems to think it's all right for him to attack them. And in class, if he doesn't want to do something he tells me, "you can't make me do it. If you do I'll have a bleed and it will be your fault." '

Andrew was thoroughly spoilt at home. His parents claimed they 'could do nothing with him'. They gave him anything he asked for and let him do whatever he wanted, because they felt guilty about his condition; and whenever they tried to say 'no' he would threaten them with a bleed. This frightened them so much that they always backed off. Andrew's haemophilia had become an extremely effective weapon, which eventually contributed to the break-up of his parents' marriage.

A few guidelines might help you to avoid the 'weapon trap':

- Give clear, direct messages about behaviour from an early age.

- Try not to shriek or shout when your toddler refuses to co-operate. Simply restate the position calmly, quietly, but with loving firmness. Even a very young child can sense whether or not you mean what you say.

- Agree with your partner on a code of behaviour, or your child will find ways to play you off against each other: 'But Mummy said I could . . .'

- Praise your child's co-operation and pay less heed to negative behaviour, for if it merits too much attention it will be seen as rewarding and then repeated often.

I know how difficult and painful it is to pretend that you are ignoring your child's display of temper. It is so tempting to 'give in', to temporarily stop all the noise and tears, to allay the fear that your frustrated child is going to get hurt. Yet once it is clearly understood that tantrums do not achieve the desired effect they cease to be a powerful tool. Nathan once kicked the wall in temper, shouting, 'I'll give myself a bleed!' Looking at his determined little face I felt my stomach lurch. I felt sick with fear but knew I must resist the temptation to give in. And he's never had a bleed as a result of temper. So don't weaken: you'll have a happier child in the end.

Growing awareness

Your child's attitude to others stems from a good or poor self-image and that image depends on you.

Dorothy Law Holte expresses this beautifully in *A Life in Your Hands*: -

If a child lives with criticism, he learns to condemn,
If a child lives with hostility, he learns to fight,
If a child lives with ridicule, he learns to be shy,
If a child lives with shame, he learns to feel guilty,
If a child lives with tolerance, he learns to be patient,
If a child lives with encouragement, he learns confidence,
If a child lives with praise, he learns to appreciate,
If a child lives with fairness, he learns justice,
If a child lives with security, he learns to have faith,
If a child lives with approval, he learns to like himself,
If a child lives with acceptance and friendship, he learns to find love in the world.

A sense of humour

Everybody needs a sense of the ridiculous, for nothing throws a situation into better perspective than seeing the funny side of it. And the physical act of laughing - a hearty belly laugh -is beneficial: it relaxes muscles, releases tension and strengthens your ability to cope. So don't miss the lighter moments of living with haemophilia. Share a family joke about the condition - in time you'll have a few. Listen to your child's comments - they can sometimes be amusing. A doctor was tapping his fingers on my son's chest during a medical examination in the children's ward. 'There's no-one in, you know,' Nathan said.

On another occasion, after a similar examination, Nathan studied the doctor's serious expression and said, 'Am I still alive?' Even a painful bleed couldn't dampen Nathan's sense of fun. We made him laugh and he made us laugh. Resting on his hospital bed he peered at the selection of drinks on the trolley before deciding: 'Please can I have hot chocolate with two hundred spoons of sugar?' And as he got older, 'be careful, one scratch and you'll bleed to death!' became a family joke.

Brothers and sisters

However much you try to be fair, brothers or sisters of your haemophilic child are bound to feel tinges of jealousy. This is so whatever the problem - Down's syndrome, asthma, haemophilia - because there are inevitably times when the affected child requires a lot of attention. Unlike adults, children see the person rather than the condition.

Children react in different ways depending on their personalities. In our family, Rachel's jealousy was expressed openly. She would throw a tantrum if she felt Nathan was getting too much attention. Benjamin, however, was more reserved emotionally. I can only recall one occasion when, aged ten, he clearly expressed his sense of unfairness. Wistfully watching the specially chartered Jumbo Jet taxiing along the runway on its return from a flight for nominated disabled or needy children, Nathan among them, Benjamin said quietly, almost to himself, 'I wish *I* had haemophilia.' Sadly, this treat was one to which brothers and sisters had not been invited.

Where a child has a disability, talent or stands out in any way, other children in the family occasionally feel excluded. Yet these times can be weathered provided each child feels valued, loved and special. Good, close relationships are still possible providing you recognise that every child in the family needs to feel special, needs sometimes to have your undivided attention and so long as you consistently try to apply the same rules to your haemophilic child as to the others.

When Rachel was eleven years she said: 'When I'm at school people come up to me and say, "What's the matter with your little brother?" I say, he's got haemophilia. So then they say, "What's haem-o-philia?" They can't even pronounce it right sometimes. And I say, it's when you haven't got all your Factor VIII, which is a clotting factor. Then they say, "What's a clotting factor?" and I have to explain it all. And they always want to see inside my SOS bracelet, they think it's some sort of secret watch. I've got mild haemophilia, but people mostly don't understand what haemophilia is, so sometimes when I get cuts they start panicking.

'I'm very close to Nathan, but sometimes we do have squabbles. We don't really take notice of his haemophilia or mine. We just play like normal friends. But when Nathan says, "My foot's hurting." I think, Oh no, not again! Who am I going to play with? Because I don't have such a close relationship with my other brothers as I do with Nathan. 'I get very jealous of him sometimes when he's in hospital -the chatter is all about Nathan and I don't get a look in. 'After a bleed, or if he has to go into hospital, he often gets into a bad mood and I get fed up with him.

'But once I went to hospital with Nathan to comfort him, because he was going to have an injection. I wanted to see what happened and Nathan wanted me there. The doctor picked up a sharp needle and began to put it in Nathan's arm. You could see by Nathan's expression that it was hurting and I could feel that pain going through me as the needle went into his arm; it was just as if it was going into my own arm. After the injection I hugged Nathan as if I was saying -1 love you and I'm glad you're my brother.'

And Simon, at the age of fourteen, said: 'If you have a brother with haemophilia you sort of wake up in the middle of the night and there's all this rushing around. You just think to yourself Oh, this is all routine stuff. I've woken up at three o'clock in the morning and found Mum rushing around - it just seems normal to me, whereas in another family without haemophilia it wouldn't be normal. 'But there are disadvantages to having a brother with haemophilia - like you couldn't teach him rugby tactics. Apart from the rugby though we don't think of Nathan as anything but a normal little boy.

'I like doing some things with Nathan like having water fights. I like getting him really soaked and I know it can't do him any harm. 'Sometimes I get jealous of Nathan, I don't know why because I wouldn't like to go to hospital and have all these injections or go for regular checkups. I mean it would be all right missing school, but I don't think it would be much fun with all the injections and having to live with this and also missing out on some games that I really enjoy. Maybe it's because of all the attention he gets with people saying, "Ah poor Nathan he's had a bleed, we must be really kind to him."'

Haemophilia takes a back seat

The haemophilic child is a child within a family. And for the family to be a happy, close unit each member must be able to give love and feel lovable. Once the initial shock of diagnosis is over and you know more about haemophilia you can begin to make sure that it does not dominate family life.
Any child's disability, although important, is only one of many aspects of daily living. And your view of it will influence not only the affected child but also the entire family. So it's important to see it in proper perspective. Feelings of guilt about haemophilia can lead you to overprotect your child. And when this happens brothers and sisters get unintentionally neglected and resent the haemophilic child who has the 'lion's share' of attention.

CHAPTER NINE

Teenager to Adult

A normal teenager

Ask any parent who has a teenager and they will probably tell you at length how difficult adolescence is. This is the case for every teenager, not just one with a blood disorder. As a parent, you may wonder at this stage where you went wrong when the child you thought you knew starts behaving in a way that seems out of character. Television characters such as Kevin the Teenager, although taken to extremes, are ones that many parents can readily recognise from living with their own teenagers.

But adolescence is as difficult for your child as it is for you. It is a time of dramatic physical change, a growing desire to be independent, establishing their own identity and an awareness of a world that is bigger and less safe than the environment they are familiar with... all this against a background of peer, media, school and parental pressures...As a parent, it is hard to stand back. But the more pressure you exert, the more your teenager is likely to rebel. Keep the lines of communication open and try not to be judgemental

It is easy to forget that we were all once teenagers and survived to emerge into adulthood as the responsible, rational people we like to think we are. If you have prepared the ground in earlier childhood, providing a loving, secure environment where your child felt valued and established good communication between you, there is no reason why your child should not develop into an adult you will be proud of.

Just as a caterpillar becomes a larva before emerging into butterfly-hood, so a child must go through the transitional period of adolescence before becoming a fully-fledged adult. Teenagers are not a species apart despite the fact that sometimes they and we regard them in that light. A blood disorder is just one more factor to be taken into account.

Self image

Teenagers are very conscious of the way they look, dress, behave and interact with others. Your sensitivity towards your child at this stage of life is extremely important. Being introspective, easily hurt and self-critical, the teenager tries to be self-protective. This defensiveness can be misinterpreted by adults as selfishness, moodiness, hostility or rudeness…

This is where it is vital to keep open the channels of communication. Reassure without being patronising, allow plenty of personal space and privacy but make it clear you are available when needed. Having haemophilia can make a teenager feel different. There may be resentment at still being dependent on adults for treatment if they are not already self-infusing. It enhances the feeling of still being a child and can lead to feelings of isolation.

The Haemophilia Society runs an Award Scheme for achievements of young people with blood disorders. Giving genuine praise whenever merited works for all ages, including teenagers as long as it doesn't sound patronising. Shouting or losing your temper is counter-productive and makes everyone feel bad.

Fitting in with the crowd

Most teenagers feel a powerful need to belong to and be accepted by a group of their own age. They worry about being an outsider for any reason. Some may try to hide their haemophilia, afraid that if others find out they may be bullied for something that makes them appear different. The opinions of people of their own age are far more important to them than those of their parents. This is not to say that they no longer respect your views – rather, they are learning to form their own ideas and opinions about life.

Rather than talk too much on his behalf I encouraged Nathan, from a very early age, to talk with and ask questions of doctors, nurses and other adults as well as speaking freely about his haemophilia with anyone who was interested in his condition. Perhaps this is part of the reason that, once he became a teenager, whilst not mentioning his condition unless the situation warranted it, he never felt a need to keep it hidden. It also helped to develop his social skills. At the time, my sole intention was to keep him involved to prevent boredom. Fortunately, it had a positive spin-off later on! Some teenagers with a blood disorder prefer not to associate with similarly affected people of their own age. Others feel happier identifying with them; your local support group is a good starting point.

Carriers

Our daughter Rachel is one of a minority of carriers of haemophilia classed as 'symptomatic'. This was diagnosed after a blood test at five years of age at my request. Today, such a test is routinely carried out at three or four years of age on a young girl where it is known that haemophilia is in the family.

A particularly low level of Factor VIII may indicate that a girl is a symptomatic carrier. This means there is a possibility that without treatment excessive bleeding may occur following such occasions as dental or other surgery, if a bone is broken and during menstruation. Medical identification can and should, be worn. Body-contact sports are best avoided. Aspirin in any form must never be taken.

Being labelled a 'symptomatic carrier' can cause confusion. It may lead to some doctors not acknowledging that a girl has haemophilia. A preferred description nowadays is 'a person with mild haemophilia'. Knowing early on that your daughter is a carrier means that it need not come as a shock during teenage years. You can talk about the need for a prescribed drug to prevent heavy bleeding during periods at an age where a mother would normally discuss such subjects with her daughter - before puberty - in a manner appropriate to her maturity and understanding.

Rachel says of her teenage years, 'I felt special.' She had always known of her carrier status and although she suffered from heavy periods, alleviated by prescribed medication, she has so far had no other symptoms. Her known carrier status put her on a level with Nathan in her eyes and helped to alleviate some of the jealousy she felt.

However, Rachel found, as many symptomatic carriers do, that some doctors did not believe that she had a bleeding disorder. If this is a problem that affects you, talk to staff at your Haemophilia Centre, who will have experience of girls in this situation. They can give advice and can put you in touch with others in a similar position. Where a girl could be a carrier of haemophilia it is important to bring her up with the awareness of this possibility and an understanding of the implications so that she will have the necessary awareness when she has children of her own. A DNA analysis can be carried out on a blood sample at around sixteen years when she is able to give her informed consent. Counselling will be given by an experienced member of staff about the feelings she may experience if the result is positive.

Transferring to an adult centre

Transfer takes place sometime during the teenage years, in hospitals where adults and children are treated separately. This can be an anxious time for the teenager and for parents. They have come to know and trust the staff in the children's centre so a move at this point can be a major upheaval.

Staff in centres are aware of this and, whilst each centre has its own arrangements, it is usual for staff from the adult centre to visit and get to know the family well before the changeover takes place. Sometimes, where there are several children due to transfer, staff from both centres will hold a 'getting to know you' social event. At the adult centre, teenagers are gradually encouraged to consult with staff without a parent being present. This gives an opportunity for them raise subjects that might be difficult to discuss with parents as well as giving a growing sense of independence.

Taking risks

There is a fine balance to be found in early years between allowing a child to take some calculated risks and setting boundaries without stifling them. In the long term this will pay off. One notable feature of teenagers is that they test limits. This often involves taking risks. Eager to explore their rapidly expanding horizons, they are drawn into a culture that includes alcohol, sex, drugs, tobacco, cars and motorbikes…

The risks here are well known and hopefully you will have discussed them with your child long before they become an issue.

Finding your own limitations involves some risk taking. It is a normal part of life. Some excesses often occur before these limits are discovered and the teenager becomes a responsible individual. There are additional risks for someone with haemophilia. Alcohol and soft drugs anaesthetise the body, meaning that bleeds can fail to be noticed early on and treatment delayed. A fall when under the influence or involvement in a fight have obvious risks…

A haemophilia nurse specialist told me that after showing and explaining the results of a liver test during a six-monthly review to a habitual teenager drinker, he vastly reduced his alcohol intake from fear of the not-to-distant consequences.

Like any other teenager, Nathan took risks, having occasional falls as a result of drinking with his friends; and he once wrote off a car (not as a result of drink!).

Despite all our warnings and advice, like most people he needed to learn from the consequences of his actions.

None of us learns from another's experience! However, sympathetic handling by staff at our Centre greatly helped him to develop a greater respect for his body.

Compliance

Self-infusion in the early teenage years will have given a boy personal control over his treatment. Not wanting to be different from others, a teenager with haemophilia may decide to ignore his condition, particularly if he has few or no bleeds whilst on prophylaxis. Preaching at him won't help. The main response is likely to be, 'It's my body..!' If this happens he is far more likely to listen to the advice of staff at his Centre than to his parents. The most powerful cure for non-compliance with treatment is probably the pain and immobility endured from leaving bleeds too long untreated.

Employment

Some employers may be dismayed at the idea of taking on a person with haemophilia. Many others, once they understand the nature of the condition are sympathetic about any difficulties of a particular person with haemophilia. When Nathan, aged sixteen, applied for a part-time job at a fast-food restaurant, asked about his condition he calmly explained that it wasn't a problem - he would just sometimes have to give himself an injection. And he got the job.

In the past, because of poor school attendance, many careers were out of reach for people with haemophilia. They lacked the necessary qualifications. Nowadays, people with haemophilia are only excluded from the Armed Forces. Realistically, difficulties in employment prospects at present for everyone make academic qualifications an important priority for any student. With modern treatment facilities today a person with haemophilia usually stands the same educational chances as the non-affected. The Haemophilia Society can give up-to-date advice.

The opposite sex

As a parent you are in the best position to know when to talk with your haemophilic son or carrier daughter about how haemophilia is passed on and how they feel about talking to a future partner about it. Until a relationship becomes more than 'just friends', any decision about whether to tell friends of the same or opposite sex about haemophilia or carrier status is an entirely personal matter and deserves respect. But once it becomes more serious, it is only fair that information is shared with a partner including implications for the future.

Safe sex is an obvious responsible measure to take in any serious relationship. An unwanted pregnancy is further complicated by the issues surrounding haemophilia. Some Comprehensive Care Centres have facilities to give counselling in plain language, which will help to answer any questions and allay any fears.

Going on holiday

Going on holiday, whether in the UK or abroad, is not a problem today for someone with haemophilia. Until a boy has begun self-infusion a parent trained to inject would accompany him on a school trip. When the time comes for independent travel the adolescent needs to take account of the amount of Factor to be taken, storage conditions and proximity of the nearest haemophilia centre. A MedicAlert bracelet or pendant is internationally recognised and gives the necessary information (The Green Card, though useful, has probably by now ended up in a washing machine!).

For overseas travel a consultant's note for Customs, holiday insurance (consult the Society for policies that cover haemophilia) and for Europe an E111 form are also essential. The Haemophilia Society is hoping to introduce adventure holidays for older teenagers.

Letting go

Giving responsibility of the condition to your child is a gradual process, which culminates in total control on leaving home – often harder for the parent than the child. But if your child feels ready to go, he probably is. And he is certainly demonstrating a willingness to accept responsibility. Before Nathan left for University, he checked that there was a fridge in which to store his Factor VIII. Treatment equipment would be locked away in his room. He phoned the nearest Haemophilia Centre and set off wearing his MedicAlert. It was several weeks before we stopped waiting for daily phone calls and began to trust that he would cope well on his own.

CHAPTER TEN

Winning Through

Trying to adjust

To continue my personal story: when Nathan was first diagnosed with haemophilia, despite persistent efforts to come to terms with it, I still found it difficult to accept that my little son had something seriously wrong with him. And although I had found out a great deal about his condition I was terrified of Nathan hurting himself. I desperately wanted to protect him from harm.

I froze whenever Nathan hurtled towards me. And I'd plead with him as he struggled off my lap, 'Please don't run, darling...'But his mischievous look dared me to run after him. His eyes shone with excitement before he rushed off again squealing with delight. To him this was simply another of Mummy's games.

What if he stumbled and fell? Of course there were times when he did. And the sick, sinking sensation inside me as I kissed him better stayed with me for hours, remained until I realised that he did not automatically have a bleed whenever he tumbled.

Each time I renewed my determination not to panic. A couple of weeks after the diagnosis, one of the GPs in our local practice rang me. 'I'm so sorry Marie,' he said, 'It must have been a terrible shock.' His sympathy triggered the now familiar silent flow of tears. 'There's someone I'd like you to meet,' he continued, 'Brian's ten years old and he's got severe haemophilia, like Nathan. I hardly ever see him nowadays because his mother injects him at home. Shall I suggest she phones you?'

I met her and, listening to the matter-of-fact way she talked about haemophilia, I began to feel more hopeful for Nathan's future. Here was somebody who had been through the same sort of hell as I had and learned to smile again, to cope so well that she could sit chatting without so much as a glance towards the garden where Brian seemed to be competing with Simon, my eldest, in a tree-climbing contest. And then Brian came into the kitchen. 'Mum, I've got a bleed in my ankle.' I looked at him. Fear washed over me. This was a situation I would have to face many times with Nathan...

A calm voice broke through my jumbled thoughts. 'Would you like to watch me inject him?' I was tempted to refuse. I couldn't bear the thought of watching a mother inflicting pain on her own child, knowing that one day I might have to do the same thing. But I was intensely curious to see how she was going to deal with this situation and how Brian would react. Neither of them seemed perturbed at the prospect of what to me seemed like a dreadful ordeal. In fact Brian and his Mum chatted normally as she meticulously prepared for the intravenous injection.

'I know it looks complicated,' she said, 'but it soon becomes automatic, like driving a car.' Brian placed his arm on the table and didn't even a flinch as his mother slid the thin needle into his vein. My stomach tightened and I had a strong urge to leave the room.

I had nothing but admiration for both of them but at that moment I knew with certainty that I would never be able to do this for Nathan, however much I wanted to. I was left with mixed feelings after their visit. Strong, healthy, athletic-looking Brian was living proof that it is perfectly possible for a haemophilic child to live normally; but perhaps that was because his mother was a stronger character, more able to cope than ever I would be...Nevertheless, I made a conscious effort to curb my anticipation of Nathan's every movement, to allow him the freedom to play and to limit my stream of 'don'ts. 'I even began to relax a little, began to enjoy some of the time we spent together. And then one Saturday morning, after Nathan had used the potty I went to empty it. One brief look at the contents made me recoil in horror- his urine was bright red. My finger trembled as I dialled the surgery number. 'Nathan's wee is red,' I told the doctor, speaking far too quickly.

He sent us to hospital. I found it difficult to concentrate on the road during the half-hour drive, with Nathan whimpering in the back of the car... Crying inside, I held Nathan's hand, stroked his forehead, kissed his face and whispered comforting words as the paediatrician tried to pull back the foreskin on his penis. Nathan cried bitterly. I felt so inadequate, so helpless. If only I could take away his pain!

The doctor gently persisted, finally managing to retract the foreskin after smearing it liberally with anaesthetic cream. 'Balanitis,' she announced. 'Inflammation of the penis. It can happen to anybody. Nothing to worry about.' No injection was necessary so we returned home with instructions to give Nathan salt baths twice daily for the next few days.

He recovered quickly and soon forgot this incident that had seemed so frightening, but inside me it was added to the pent-up store of emotion that would soon overflow completely.

Baby Benjamin

My fourth child was almost due when I went for an ultra-sound scan. 'I can't see anything to suggest it's a boy,' said the gynaecologist carefully studying the result. 'But of course, I can't guarantee that you'll have a girl.' Nevertheless I felt reassured and - apart from a small nagging doubt during the remaining weeks of my pregnancy -1 was convinced that Rachel would soon have her longed-for sister. When my waters broke in the early hours of May 8th we set off for the hospital leaving my husband's aunt and the children asleep.

We spent that day in the labour room enjoying our first real respite since the diagnosis three months previously. We read, listened to music and relaxed. But by the evening doctors decided to speed up my well-spaced contractions.

Soon after, amid powerful contractions, I felt a strong urge to push. 'It's a little boy,' the midwife said quietly. She knew why I desperately wanted a girl.

Every part of me hurt. She must have got it wrong. This couldn't be happening Les cradled our baby son, but I buried my face in the pillow. 'Look at him, darling, he's beautiful,' Les said. I turned my head slowly. Les leaned forward to kiss me, bringing the tiny body in a white blanket close to my face. A searing pain shot through me. An overwhelming tide of emotion swept through my body. I felt utterly helpless, completely unable to prevent its release. All the unexpressed emotion about Nathan's haemophilia flooded out of me in a seemingly unending rush.

I could hear a primitive, piercing sound like the wailing of a wounded animal. I was dimly aware that it came from me but could do nothing to control it. It took two tranquillising injections to calm me. I breast-fed Benjamin . . . but I felt nothing. For the next few months I lived in a twilight world. Drugged, apathetic and only vaguely aware of what was happening around me, I fed my baby whenever he cried but did little else. Sometimes a small curly head nuzzled against my arm, a soft hand gently stroked my cheek. 'Mummy tired,' Nathan would say.

Social Services provided a home help to cover most of the time Les was teaching but there were still hours when Nathan, left to his own devices, was able to develop the sort of independence that is normal for a two-year-old - without the hindrance of a stair gate, he not only learned how to manoeuvre the stairs but to go up and down them freely, he chose where he played, used scissors, helped himself to any biscuits he fancied . . . In fact, by the time I emerged from my post-natal depression he was an extremely capable little boy, though I shudder to think of the many dangers he had to avoid in getting to that stage.

Complacency

Coming out of my depression was like surfacing from a deep, dark pit. I began to notice, to appreciate, love and enjoy my beautiful six-month-old baby and take pride in confident, happy Nathan. We'd bath Benjamin and laugh as his chubby little legs kicked vigorously, splashing us with water. Afterwards Nathan would sprinkle the soft wriggly body with powder and help me to dress him. I'd tickle them both and we'd all be rolling on the floor helpless with laughter. Tests soon after birth had shown that Benjamin did not have haemophilia and although there were still moments when it hurt me to look at Nathan's lovely face and remember that he did, my love for him seemed heightened by his vulnerability. Anyway, how could I resist such a warm-hearted, handsome, friendly child?

I began to realise that whole days had passed without the need for any injections. And once I'd made the decision to live 'one day at a time' I could say as I kissed my sleeping son, 'Today was a good day.' Then as days stretched into weeks and months without any of the predicted bleeds, we began to wonder if the doctors had somehow made a dreadful mistake.

'You see . . . he's all right - they've got it wrong,' said an aunt. Nevertheless, I often read Dick Bruna's Children's Haemophilia Book to Nathan, gradually familiarising him with the condition that deep down I suspected he did have, that made me feel so terribly sad whenever anybody mentioned it. But when almost three years had passed without mishap we triumphantly presented Nathan for his six-monthly check-up. Even the doctor's warning against complacency could not dampen our enthusiasm about Nathan's bleed-free existence. We relaxed our vigilance, bought him a tricycle, let him live normally.

'He leads a charmed life,' said Les. Then, one Saturday morning, shortly before his fifth birthday, the snow fell. Nathan came in from the garden complaining that his foot hurt. But when I examined it there was no sign of swelling and Nathan's 'It only hurts a bit' reassured me. However, by teatime Nathan's ankle was swollen, he couldn't walk and was trying hard to hold back the tears. Annoyed with myself for doing nothing sooner, I rang the duty G.P. When he arrived, he gently pressed the swelling and rotated Nathan's foot. 'How did it happen?' he asked.

Nathan couldn't remember injuring it. 'He's sprained it; we'll strap it up for a few days. Keep him off his feet,' said the doctor. 'He doesn't need to go to hospital?' I queried. 'No, it's just a sprain,' he said. I expressed my relief to Les that night when he rang - he was away on a weekend study course. But during the night a tearful voice woke me. 'My foot's hurting terribly Mummy.'

I settled Nathan in bed beside me and rang the doctor again. 'Nathan's in a lot of pain.' I said. 'He will be - sprains are painful. Give him some Calpol. I'll drop by in the morning.' The Calpol made little difference to the pain. I held Nathan close for hours while he cried.   And when eventually he slept, it was my turn to cry.

The next morning Nathan's ankle was less painful. The doctor advised further rest and the problem seemed to resolve itself after a few days. But two weeks later Nathan's ankle began to swell painfully once more. This time worry and instinct persuaded me to ring Doctor Scott, a paediatrician at the West Suffolk Hospital, twenty miles away.

'Bring him in now,' she said. Feeling extremely dejected I drove Nathan to the hospital. I forced back the tears as Nathan chattered away, not wanting him to see my distress. Trying not to alarm him I talked to him about the injection he would be given to make the pain go away. 'Will it hurt?' he asked. 'Yes, it will a bit but the injection will take away the pain in your ankle.' 'All right then Mummy, but will you stay with me?' he asked anxiously. 'I promise I won't leave you,' I reassured him. 'And if it hurts you can squeeze my hand as hard as you like.' Nathan was injected with cryoprecipitate and we stayed overnight in hospital. The next morning the consultant paediatrician examined Nathan. 'I wish your doctor wouldn't treat bleeds by just leaving them,' she said crossly.

Time for school

After a few further bleeds into Nathan's ankle joint the paediatrician advised a short spell in a wheelchair. He was understandably self-conscious as I wheeled him into the school grounds for his first full day at school. 'I don't want to go to school.' he said, then pointing to a child in the playground he exclaimed, 'Look, she's laughing at me.' My attempt to explain that she wasn't even looking his way failed to comfort him. However, when the bell rang and his teacher, who already knew what to expect, wheeled Nathan to the classroom, his face brightened as he recognised some of his friends from nursery school. My final anxious glimpse through the window was of Nathan smiling and chatting with them.

Children who knew him always accepted Nathan in or out of a wheelchair, with or without a bleed. To them he was just Nathan, they enjoyed his company. And happily he has always made friends easily. After that first day he never showed any reluctance at the school gate.

A series of bleeds

Although Nathan spent the morning of his fifth birthday in hospital on account of yet another bleed into his left ankle, he was home in time for his party in the afternoon. He brought with him a present from the paediatrician which he proudly demonstrated - the syringe with multiple adaptors was a marvellous water pistol. A couple of days later Nathan had a sore throat and a high temperature. The doctor diagnosed tonsillitis and put him on antibiotics, which seemed to take effect. However, he was nearing the end of the course when early one morning he uttered a strangled sort of sound.

Les ran fast to see what had happened and by the time I reached the landing he was already on his way back. His face was white. 'There's blood dripping from Nathan's mouth,' he said. At first we thought that Nathan might have bitten his tongue or the inside of his mouth, but after a quick inspection I realised that the blood must be coming from his throat.

Surprisingly, Nathan did not seem unduly concerned as I cleaned his face with a damp sponge and gave him a towel to catch the slow drips that I could do nothing to stop.

'It's all right Nathan,' I said, 'Just stay there; I'll be back in a minute.'

But it wasn't right. Shaking from head to foot with panic I rang my G.P. 'Nathan's bleeding from the throat and I can't stop it,' I shouted.

'Calm down, Marie, ring an ambulance and get him to hospital.' The doctor's even tone steadied me a little.

While Les coped with Benjamin who had woken crying, I rushed around trying frantically to collect my thoughts and necessary items for our hospital trip. The ambulance attendant wrapped Nathan in a blanket and carried him out into the misty grey morning. Was it perhaps the calm, gentle way he talked to Nathan that stopped the relentless dripping during the journey to hospital? It reminded me of what I had read about Rasputin talking calmly to the little Prince Alexei.

On arrival at the hospital a doctor we had never seen before studied Nathan's hospital notes before examining him. 'Hello Natman,' she said, obviously unfamiliar with his name. That cut the tension . . . even Nathan laughed. 1985 was a difficult year. From April to July Nathan bled a total of nine times into his left ankle. I'm sure our old Austin Allegro knew its own way to the hospital.

The staff on the children's ward were consistently friendly and welcoming. We even reached the stage where Nathan was allowed to choose his bed for the night!

Each time he had to stay I would remain too, returning home before Les left for work. And I would collect him in the late afternoon, after the consultant's ward round, with verbal instructions regarding night time splinting and progressive steps to full mobilisation.

Should we cancel our August seaside holiday? Finally we decided that we all desperately needed the break. The times when the needle would not enter a vein immediately were the hardest. Nathan's veins were tiny and difficult to locate. He always lay very still but his distress made my stomach churn.

On one occasion when the doctor failed to pierce the vein at the fourth attempt, I said testily, 'Please get someone else to do it.' To my surprise and to his credit he agreed. As always, the brave face I put on for Nathan during his treatment disappeared as soon as I was alone.

Lulls and crises

'He's fine,' was something we quickly learned to avoid saying when anybody asked about Nathan. For almost always, Fate would reward such complacency with a bleed, often, strangely, on a Sunday. But life eased considerably. Nathan had several bleed-free months at a time and we were able to devote more time to our other children who were beginning to pine for attention. I was no longer startled whenever the phone rang during school hours, thinking that the call inevitably concerned Nathan. And our new-found ability to 'let go' gave Nathan the freedom to learn his own limitations, to learn to live with his condition which was, after all, only a part of his busy existence - playing with friends, cycling and attending the Beavers group (a pre-cub scouts organisation) were far more important to Nathan.

We now coped far more confidently and calmly with familiar bleeds into his ankle, big toe joints and leg muscles. But occasionally we ran into crises that reminded us never to underestimate the potential seriousness of any bleed.

'Experience teaches slowly and at the cost of mistakes' (J.A. Froude). Like the time when the middle finger of Nathan's right hand swelled slightly and was just a bit painful. Nathan had an injection of cryoprecipitate the first time it happened. But a few days later when it recurred we agreed with the G.P. that it was safe to adopt a 'wait and see' approach. Two nights later only a strong sedative calmed Nathan who was screaming with the pain. I arranged to take him directly to hospital- the time was 10.30 pm.

His finger was not only swollen and discoloured but he was unable to bend it. 'We'll keep an eye on him overnight,' said the paediatrician after the injection. 'It's possible that the blood supply to that finger could be compromised.' Throughout the injections and the weeks of physiotherapy that followed I vowed never again to think: 'Well. . . it's only a finger.'

'Normal' family life

When we found out that Nathan had haemophilia I never thought that we could ever be a 'normal' family again. But by the time he was five, we had already learnt to see beyond the condition to the vivacious, happy, responsive child who added so much to our family life. We decided to have another baby. During this pregnancy I knew and accepted that I had a chance of having another child with haemophilia. I also knew that if that happened we would be able to cope. I refused the repeated offer of tests in the first few months. 'Don't you want to know if your baby is a haemophiliac?' asked the gynaecologist. But I had no intention of jeopardising my pregnancy. After a scan at twenty-five weeks the doctor said, 'Everything is fine except that it's a boy.'

I now had a one in two chance of my baby having haemophilia. Seeing my distress the doctor continued, 'You must decide what you want to do about the pregnancy.' The shock of his words stopped my tears. Looking at him directly I made no attempt to conceal my anger. 'I have no intention of having a termination.' Driving home I thought of the apparently healthy baby moving freely around inside me. I'd seen him with my own eyes on the large screen. I was stunned at the suggestion that his life be ended a few months before his birth date.

When Joel was born in May 1986, a few weeks after Nathan's sixth birthday, the whole family was delighted. And tests proved that he did not have haemophilia. By the time Nathan was eight I had managed to allow him to live, for the most part, the normal life of any boy of his age and join in the same activities as his friends.

We made the same behaviour rules for him as for our other children. We all had to adjust to the nuisance value of hospital trips, but learned quickly to combine most of them with a family shopping expedition or a visit to the park. And soon I would inject Nathan at home, which would make life easier. Our five children played and quarrelled like children in other families - each child was different, each one important.

AIDS rumours

In November 1986 rumours that Nathan might have AIDS were circulating among mothers of children who attended the same school. I first heard about them outside a local supermarket, late one Friday evening. 'Do you know that people are talking about you?' my friend said. 'They're saying that the headmaster rang you to ask if Nathan had AIDS and that as you refused to tell him he intends to consult a doctor for the truth.' 'Perhaps I shouldn't have told you,' she added anxiously, seeing the effect of her words. 'Thank you, I'm glad you did,' I said.

Shopping forgotten I headed straight for home.

'Whatever's the matter?' Les said.

'People are implying that Nathan's got AIDS.' My words shook him. A year before we had been prepared for repercussions locally when a haemophilic schoolboy in Hampshire, who was HIV positive, had made headline news. Parents had withdrawn their children from his school until Doctor Tony Pinching, an AIDS expert, had reassured them that all their fears were groundless. When I heard this news I went cold. Everybody in the neighbourhood knew about Nathan's haemophilia. Would they now shun him? For the next few weeks I worriedly scanned people's faces and waited . . . but when Nathan's friends still played in our house and he continued to be welcomed at theirs I relaxed.

Then suddenly, unexpectedly, AIDS hysteria spread to our Suffolk village. 'We'd better ring the press before they approach us,' Les suggested. Fear turned to anger. Nathan's antibody status was our own affair. Who else had the right to know whether or not he carried the AIDS virus? But some people would infer from our silence that Nathan was antibody-positive and others would conclude that he had AIDS.

To protect my child I felt I had to speak out. I rang the editor of a local free weekly newspaper who accepted my article which contained the negative results of blood tests on Nathan for the HIV virus. When a regional newspaper repeated the story a free-lance journalist for a national paper rang me for a quote. And when I refused he threatened to write his own version. Rather than be misquoted or have the story sensationalised, I contacted the medical editor of The Independent newspaper who agreed to publish my own account. Tension faded, many mothers expressed their support and the cruel rumours stopped.

One evening, remembering how when I was seven children had taunted me in the playground about the fact that I was adopted, I said to Nathan: 'Do children ever ask if you have a disease?' 'Yes,' he said, 'they often say "What nasty disease have you got Nathan?"'

I swallowed hard. 'And what do you tell them?' I said quietly. 'I say I've got haemophilia,' Nathan replied.

Learning to cope

'If a man carries his own lantern, he need not fear darkness.' (Hasidic saying)

Nathan cannot remember a time when he didn't know about his haemophilia. And his acceptance of the condition and its treatment helped us to adjust. He even made me feel useful during injections:

'Mummy, tell me when the needle goes in and when it comes out,' he said once he was able to talk in sentences. The occasional 'It's not fair!' expressed his frustration at being restricted after a bleed into a lower limb, then he found an alternative equally rewarding activity, or he bargained his way back to mobility: 'Let me go up the stairs just this once, then you can carry me down,' he said with an irresistible twinkling in his eyes. Years of living with haemophilia proved valuable -Les and I developed and matured on a personal level and we learned to value our children . . . each one is vulnerable in a different way. By the age of eight Nathan was a self-assured, warm, loving child who trusted and respected our judgement. He did not hesitate when I suggested that I learn to inject him now that his bleeds were treated with Factor VIII concentrate. 'When will you start?' he asked eagerly.

In his own words

I asked Nathan, when he was eight, what it was like to have a bleed. 'When I get a bleed it starts with pins and needles and the pain sort of gradually builds up. It starts to get worse if you leave it. I get a stabbing pain and it hurts a lot. Sometimes, when there's something exciting going on, I don't want to tell you when I've got a pain but I do anyway because otherwise the swelling increases and the pain gets much worse. I get a lot of problems with my big toe, but I can go for weeks without having a bleed. Then it just suddenly happens.

'The worst bleed I've ever had was probably in my finger. I was in a lot of pain and I couldn't bend it. That bleed started when I was tidying up my bedroom. When the pain increased my hand started aching, but at least I could still run around. If I tense up when I have an injection it gets very painful and once a doctor tried five times before the needle went in ... it hurt a lot. Having haemophilia is not as bad as it sounds because it sounds like you can't run around at all, but that isn't the case. I've got a climbing frame and I can jump around.

'When I go to hospital I think Rachel gets all upset inside. She misses me a lot because we play together. I get quite a lot of attention, which is nice. Some people say, "You nearly got AIDS didn't you?" If you don't know about haemophilia you probably think it's a dreadful disease that makes you very ill. But it's not that sort of thing. One day though I hope they find a cure for haemophilia as sometimes there's something going on that I have to miss because I've got a bleed.'

Learning to inject

A move from Suffolk to Lincoln in 1988, when Nathan was eight, provided the perfect opportunity for me to begin learning to inject him. We lived only ten minutes by car from the Haemophilia Centre at Lincoln County Hospital. And I was keen to start, to avoid the time spent driving to hospital and waiting for a doctor to carry out treatment; eager to have control over treating bleeds immediately and enjoy more time at home with the rest of the family.

Nathan's treatment had recently been changed from cryoprecipitate to freeze dried Factor VIII; I had watched it being prepared several times. The haemophilia sister- Brenda Brown- was very encouraging and her training was thorough.

Although he looked apprehensive the first time I prepared to insert the needle under medical supervision, Nathan was delighted when it slid directly into the vein. And he did not flinch when, on another occasion, I missed a vein. 'Try the other arm,' he suggested. I lined the needle up with the vein and slowly pierced his skin. We watched the blood flowing along the plastic tubing that led to the syringe. 'It's in!' he shouted triumphantly, recognising the sign of success. I released the tourniquet and we watched the liquid slowly disappear into Nathan's vein, as I pressed gently on the plunger of the syringe. Lightly as a feather, I withdrew the butterfly needle from his arm, pressed for a few minutes on the point of injection with a tiny ball of cotton wool and we exchanged smiles of relief. It was a great confidence booster for us both.

However, over the next six months, things began to go wrong. Preparing the Factor VIII was the easy part. But sometimes it would take two or three attempts for me to get the needle into his vein. Because he was small for his age, Nathan's veins were not easily visible. And although he put on a brave face I could see the pain in his eyes and cringed inwardly. On one occasion, knowing the Factor VIII had to be used within a short time once it was prepared; I had to call out the G.P. to give the injection. I felt a failure.

'Practice on me,' said Brenda, at the Haemophilia Centre.

The needle pierced her vein without difficulty.

'It's easy with you,' I protested. 'Your veins are like motorways. But Nathan's are so hard to find and when I put the needle in, the vein seems to disappear completely.'

'Persevere and you'll succeed,' she replied confidently. 'I know you can do it.' I was determined to succeed. And she was right. Before long, although I always feared missing the vein, with Nathan's encouragement and my own intense concentration, I was scoring a direct hit every time. And each time I gave Nathan a little reward and he gave me a kiss.

Early adolescence

By the age of eleven it became clear that Nathan's left ankle was a target joint. This meant several short spells in a wheelchair following a bleed to give it a chance to recover. Nathan particularly disliked having to use the wheelchair at school. He accepted that it was necessary but discarded it at the earliest opportunity. At secondary school a change of ancillary helper came as a shock to him and me. Nathan would complain many times, 'She keeps fussing over me.' Despite my visits to talk with her about his condition and encourage her to keep the supervision discreet, her over-protectiveness continued.

Nevertheless, he was never short of friends and our house was always full of happy, noisy children – our own and other people's. I used to think of haemophilia as the worst thing that could happen to a child. But during primary and early secondary school, I saw the suffering of one of Nathan's friends, Kevin, who had cystic fibrosis, often watched him struggle to breathe. I realised that the ways in which Kevin's condition affected him and his mother were far more serious than Nathan's. And at fourteen, Kevin died.

As a teacher myself I knew the importance of regular school attendance in order to avoid falling behind. So I kept his absences to a minimum and Nathan began to achieve good results, particularly in languages and music. He developed several 'crazes' like the rest of the family - remote-control car racing, CB radio and hand-held computer games, to name a few. But an enduring passion was his music. He had piano lessons alongside Benjamin and began playing the guitar.

Self-infusion

Nathan had come to rely on me injecting him and was in no hurry to begin self-treatment. Finally, during a review at the Haemophilia Centre when Nathan was sixteen, Brenda handed him an orange and said, 'I think it's about time you learned to inject yourself. Practise on this.' Sometimes it was hard to stand back and let him get on with self-treatment. I found it difficult to watch him struggling with the process so preferred to go into another room rather than try to take over or convey the tension I was feeling. I knew that just as I had had to get to grips with the whole process, it was important to let him find his way at his own pace.

It took him a while to get the hang of it but, always noted for his tenacity, he eventually succeeded. This gave him more control over his life and it gave me more freedom. Sometimes he delayed treating a bleed in favour of more interesting diversions. These times I found particularly hard, knowing from an X-ray that he already had signs of arthritis in his ankle. And there were other occasions that I only found out about much later.

Late Teens

Having four other children ensured that I did not focus too closely on Nathan's journey through adolescence. Haemophilia apart, he was in every way a normal teenager – at times rebellious, adventurous, argumentative, loving... And he couldn't wait to start driving. He passed his test at the first attempt, at seventeen and spent many happy hours with Benjamin and their friends driving round the Lincolnshire countryside, sometimes sitting and talking into the small hours, sometimes hunting ghosts in reputedly-haunted areas. He got a part-time job to pay for petrol! He joined a rock band and gained a reputation locally as a lead singer, guitarist and keyboard player. He even went round local restaurants until he got a job playing piano. He still managed to squeeze in time for schoolwork somehow.

Family of adults

For a year, at the age of twenty, Nathan lived with his girlfriend Sarah in Spain. His haematologist rang unexpectedly to tell him that a recent donor to his plasma-derived Factor VIII had died of CJD. Nathan asked him the implications. Doctor Adelman told him that although there was no proven risk of transmission through blood products, there was still a very small chance of Nathan developing the disease in twenty to thirty years. Nathan replied, 'Thanks for letting me know. Now I'll get on with the rest of my life.'

And that's just what he's doing today – and getting the maximum out of it. Les and I are proud of all five of our children. They are positive, well-balanced individuals with a high degree of self-belief. I asked each one to contribute to this book in their own way.

Joel, now eighteen, has this to say:

'I can't remember any particular incident when I realised Nathan had haemophilia. It was just general knowledge. It was the normal thing – I didn't question it. Perhaps it was part of my disposition that I accepted it. I had a happy childhood. Nathan didn't stand out much at all, to be honest. He was just my brother. From eight to sixteen I got on best with Nathan and Ben. I remember joking with Nathan about his haemophilia. It wasn't really an issue when I was younger.

'I'm no more worried about Nathan than I am about my other brothers because he's got his haemophilia under control. I've only had brief jealous moments once or twice since I started to drive and found how expensive it is. And his Mobility Allowance means he doesn't have to pay out for insurance, tax and a car. I remember telling my friends he got it for free.

'When I see Nathan now, we have in-depth chats. I don't think I've ever talked with him about haemophilia.'

Benjamin, twenty-two, writes:

'Growing up having a brother with haemophilia was in some ways difficult. Because of the frequent medical attention Nathan required I was sometimes left feeling resentful towards him because of the fact that he was getting more attention than I was. In hindsight this seems stupid but as a child I could not see it from anyone else's point of view but my own.

'I envied Nathan for the advantages his haemophilia seemed to bring him, failing to see stresses it must have caused him as well as my parents. This caused us to argue sometimes although we did generally get along. It wasn't until my late teens that we started to become closer. Being of relatively similar age we found we had increasingly more in common as we both matured and started seeing things from each other's point of view. The haemophilia is no longer an issue in the slightest and we are now best friends as well as brothers. Instead of resenting him for his disability I now respect both him and my parents for the way they have coped with it.'

Simon, thirty, says:

'Nathan is more like a mate than a brother now. When he got to eighteen it was different because we started going out and it was like going out drinking with anybody else. He acted the same as somebody who wasn't affected by haemophilia. It didn't seem to affect him at all; he did pretty much what he wanted. To him it's the same as someone who's got the flu. I mean if he has a bleed it's the same as someone going home and taking a flu capsule, except he injects. I don't think it has affected the family. How often does anybody mention his haemophilia? They don't. Only when Mum's writing the book. Nobody says "How's Nathan's haemophilia?"'

And Rachel, twenty-seven, writes:

'Each and every one of my brothers is unique. If you asked me to describe Simon, for example, I would use words such as: "Great Alan Partridge impersonator". For Joel: "Mr.Fitness", Ben: "First-class smooth talker", Nathan: "Free spirit". The only time the word 'haemophilia' comes to mind is when Mum asks for comments for her book on the subject. '"Handicapped" doesn't even feature in my thoughts about Nathan. He may not be normal in other areas such as his dress sense and be disadvantaged as far as his hairdresser is concerned but, for me, his haemophilia is a physical trait such as blood type or shoe size. That is exactly how I feel about talking about my haemophilia. I have mild haemophilia and I also carry it in my genes – but that's just a part of my body. People love labelling things. I fall into an infinite number of categories and "girl affected by haemophilia" is just one of them. I am Rachel.'

CHAPTER ELEVEN

The Last Word

Since Nathan, now aged twenty-four, was the inspiration for this book it is fitting that he has the final say. He made this contribution just before setting off for a holiday in Jamaica with his girlfriend Donna, with Factor VIII in his luggage and a letter from Doctor Adelman, his haematologist, to clear him through Customs.

'I've always known I have haemophilia. I've been told about it from an early age in a very factual way. For me, living with haemophilia is the same as anybody else living *their* life because it's all I've ever known. I just have to inject myself and other people don't. To an outsider it may look like a horrible thing, having to stick needles in your arm. But if that's what you've always done, you're not going to think of it as something terrible.

'My earliest memory is of going to school in a wheelchair at about four or five. I didn't want to be different from the other kids. It can be a bit frustrating when you want to be out doing things and you can't be. Having to be pushed in a chair is not something you want. I didn't have to do it very often and because I didn't feel different I didn't act any differently. So people didn't treat me differently. I was a bit nervous about Mum injecting me at first because she missed the vein a lot. But then she became proficient at it and it wasn't a problem. It was just standard routine and made life easier because I didn't have to go up to the hospital every time and it meant that when we went away we didn't have to worry where the nearest hospital was to get Factor VIII from. So there were a lot of benefits to it.

'My ancillary helper at secondary school would fuss over me and treat me as if I was a special child, which was a bit annoying. You don't want to appear different from the other kids. When you're a teenager you want to appear cool. You want to wear the newest clothes and the latest trainers. You don't want to stand out in any way that could be perceived as negative. So the fact that some woman is going around telling everyone to be careful of you obviously doesn't make you feel good. You tend to fend less for yourself if someone's doing things for you all the time. You almost play the role that you're given.

'When you're told you need an ancillary as a child and you've got this lady following you round school I think you tend to grow up a lot slower. You're treated as a child right the way through school because you've got something wrong with you.

'I think haemophilia is misunderstood by a lot of people, even some doctors. My ancillary used to talk to me as though I was a lot younger. When you're at the stage where you're forming your own opinions and working out what you think of yourself, what you can and can't do, you don't need someone constantly saying, "You can't do this and you can't do that" and, "Watch yourself when you're doing this," because that then becomes a part of how you see yourself. And because you know that you get more attention I think on reflection at school I played more on things to get attention in a subtle way. It hasn't affected my ability to make friends but socially there's still that feeling of being a bit different in a group. I tend to leave things to others and have a less pro-active attitude. That might just be me though because a lot of people are like that anyway. At school you develop the social part of yourself. I haven't got a problem with haemophilia but I think I might have been a bit different if I'd grown up without it.

'I was never bullied by other children. I'd get asked questions about haemophilia but not much because I think people worried that I was going to be sensitive about it. Luckily I had a home life that counteracted it because I was treated completely normally. I never felt any different from how you would feel in a family or close-knit situation. I would fight and play with my brothers and sister and do everything they did. If I had a bleed I would go off, have an injection, come back and carry on playing. My mum and dad were never over-protective. They would just throw in words of advice and caution. Probably at the start that was something they had to work at but they never stopped me doing anything I wanted to do. I was lucky there was nothing I passionately wanted to do that I couldn't. I suppose if a child grows up wanting a career in the armed services then it's going to be a big problem.

'As I was growing up doctors, teachers and parents looked after me. They'd say, "You need an injection," when I had a bleed. When I got older, sometimes when I wanted to go and play football and realised I had a bleed coming on, I wouldn't say anything about it because I knew I would then be told, "You can't go and play football when you've got a bleed." So I'd play football and *then* tell them I had a bleed, which obviously isn't a good thing to do.

'When I started injecting myself I began to take responsibility for my haemophilia and realised that, actually, this is my condition. But sometimes I was reckless, like all teenagers are. I took a running jump off our garage roof once when I was seventeen. I thought I'd be clever to show off to some girl there. I landed in the garden, sprained both my ankles and ended up on crutches until they got better. And I obviously had to give myself Factor VIII. I spent time at the hospital with Mum when I was young. This created a special sort of bond. And Dad as well – he used to take me out for walks to make sure I kept active.

'I've always had a very close relationship with my parents and my brothers and sister. They were taught to see my condition in the same way I do. I was never jealous of them for not having haemophilia. I think there was probably jealousy at times on their part but I got on well with them and I didn't actually notice any. They didn't treat me any differently from how they treated each other. We still had fights. Living with haemophilia now can be a bit of a hassle because I can't leave it down to everyone else. When you move out of home, you realise it's *your* problem. You've not got someone saying to you, "You'd better get that injected before you go out." At first I did leave bleeds and was a bit reckless, to be honest. When I got into my late teens there were things I would want to do, like starting Karate or something like that, so it was more difficult. I did four or five lessons of Kung Fu and I got a couple of bleeds from it. So I weighed it up and I thought, I can't really do that, it's not advisable. I think that's one thing you become more conscious of. You do think to the future a bit more.

'When you're a teenager and someone says, "When you're in your thirties you'll have to have an operation for your arthritis," you think that's never going to happen. You're never going to be that age. You don't think about getting older. But when you get into your early twenties you start to question your life. That feeling of immortality goes and you think, I *am* going to get old. My arthritis now affects me a lot more than it used to. It's not debilitating yet but it certainly does restrict me in what I can do. If I were to play football for ten or fifteen minutes my arthritis would flare up and I'd get pain in my ankle. Even walking around too much can make it hurt.

'I think the lesson I've learnt is to make sure I inject myself in time when I have a bleed. You don't want to have repeated bleeds into one joint because that can cause arthritis so you don't act over-cautious but you make sure that when you do have a bleed you inject promptly and treat yourself responsibly. Everyone has to know what their limits are in certain situations, whether they've got a disability or not. The fact that I have got a disability means that I do have to take it into account sometimes, which I do subconsciously because it's something I've been brought up with. If I'm in a situation that's likely to cause a bleed or inflame my arthritis, then I will probably back out of it unless it's something I really want to do. And then I go into it knowing what the consequences are going to be and take the necessary precautions, including giving myself an injection...

'Even now, when I get up for work and I've got a bleed in my ankle it's an annoyance, but it's not something that worries me. Haemophilia has never been an issue with my girlfriend or any of my other friends. Donna already knew about it when she first met me, because I went out with a friend of hers when I was eighteen. Donna's attitude to my haemophilia treatment is the same as mine to her clothes shopping – she needs clothes, it's just something she does. If I have to have an injection, she doesn't say, "Do you need any help?" or "Do you want me to get the sharps bin for you?" That's the best attitude anyone can have to it because if I sat down to inject myself and said, "I've got a bleed in my ankle," and she said, "Oh, do you want me to get all your stuff for you?" even that would be going too far. It's not needed. Donna is not fazed by it in the slightest. She just lets me get on with it.

'When we talked about kids she asked, "Will our kids have haemophilia?" I just said, "No, but all the girls will be carriers and our grandkids have a fifty-percent chance of having it." I've never had the situation where I've had to think, how am I going to tell someone about my haemophilia? It's never been an issue. Unless it comes up I don't really mention it. A lot of people I know don't even know I've got it. I don't mention it because it doesn't occur to me to do so. There are times I have to inject myself when a friend's there I've known for a while. I say, "I've got to give myself an injection," and they say, "What's that for?" I explain I've got haemophilia and sometimes have to give myself injections of Factor VIII, which will clot my blood and stop any internal bleeding, but that it's nothing serious. And because they don't really know anything about haemophilia they hear my attitude towards it, they see the way I act and that's their opinion of it as well, because it's the only thing they've got to go on. It's the only perception they've got of it.

'For me, having to treat haemophilia is like having to do the washing up when you've finished dinner. Everyone has to do it, they don't really want to do it but it doesn't stand out in their life. They just see it as a normal part of life. It's the way you tell it! If I pitied myself, I would tell it like that and people would pity me.

'Haemophilia has never been a problem in any workplace either.

'When I get older, if I have to have an operation on my ankle, that's just the way the cookie crumbles. I don't take unnecessary risks but I'm not over-cautious. I think what you put into your brain about your body becomes what your body *is*. If I were to worry about my haemophilia and think it was going to affect me a lot, then obviously it would.

'I think the only restrictions you have in life to do with your disability are the restrictions you place on yourself. Listen to your body, listen to yourself and do what feels right.'

Printed in the United Kingdom
by RPM Print & Design, Chichester